Cosmetic Procedures in Gynecology

Guest Editor

DOUGLAS W. LAUBE, MD, MEd

OBSTETRICS AND GYNECOLOGY CLINICS OF NORTH AMERICA

www.obgyn.theclinics.com

Consulting Editor
WILLIAM F. RAYBURN, MD, MBA

December 2010 • Volume 37 • Number 4

SAUNDERS an imprint of ELSEVIER, Inc.

W.B. SAUNDERS COMPANY

A Division of Elsevier Inc.

Elsevier, Inc. • 1600 John F. Kennedy Blvd. • Suite 1800 • Philadelphia, PA 19103-2899

http://www.theclinics.com

OBSTETRICS AND GYNECOLOGY CLINICS OF NORTH AMERICA Volume 37, Number 4
December 2010 ISSN 0889-8545, ISBN-13: 978-1-4377-2471-4

Editor: Carla Holloway
Developmental Editor: Donald Mumford

Obstetrics and Gynecology Clinics (ISSN 0889-8545) is published quarterly by Elsevier Inc., 360 Park Avenue South, New York, NY 10010-1710. Months of issue are March, June, September, and December. Periodicals postage paid at New York, NY, and additional mailing offices. Subscription price per year is $275.00 (US individuals), $474.00 (US institutions), $137.00 (US students), $331.00 (Canadian individuals), $598.00 (Canadian institutions), $201.00 (Canadian students), $402.00 (foreign individuals), $598.00 (foreign institutions), and $201.00 (foreign students). To receive student/resident rate, orders must be accompanied by name of affiliated institution, date of term, and the signature of program/residency coordinator on institution letterhead. Orders will be billed at individual rate until proof of status is received. Foreign air speed delivery is included in all *Clinics* subscription prices. All prices are subject to change without notice. POSTMASTER: Send address changes to *Obstetrics and Gynecology Clinics*, Elsevier Health Sciences Division, Subscription Customer Service, 3251 Riverport Lane, Maryland Heights, MO 63043. **Customer Service: Telephone: 1-800-654-2452 (U.S. and Canada); 314-447-8871 (outside U.S. and Canada). Fax: 314-447-8029. E-mail: journalscustomerservice-usa@elsevier.com (for print support); journalsonlinesupport-usa@elsevier.com (for online support).**

Reprints. For copies of 100 or more of articles in this publication, please contact the Commercial Reprints Department, Elsevier Inc., 360 Park Avenue South, New York, New York 10010-1710. Tel.: 212-633-3818; Fax: 212-462-1935; E-mail: reprints@elsevier.com.

Obstetrics and Gynecology Clinics of North America is also published in Spanish by McGraw-Hill Interamericana Editores S.A., P.O. Box 5-237, 06500, Mexico; in Portuguese by Reichmann and Affonso Editores, Rio de Janeiro, Brazil; and in Greek by Paschalidis Medical Publications, Athens, Greece.

Obstetrics and Gynecology Clinics of North America is covered in MEDLINE/PubMed (Index Medicus), Excerpta Medica, Current Concepts/Clinical Medicine, Science Citation Index, BIOSIS, CINAHL, and ISI/BIOMED.

Printed and bound in the United Kingdom
Transferred to Digital Print 2011

GOAL STATEMENT

The goal of *Obstetrics and Gynecology Clinics of North America* is to keep practicing physicians up to date with current clinical practice in OB/GYN by providing timely articles reviewing the state of the art in patient care.

ACCREDITATION

The *Obstetrics and Gynecology Clinics of North America* is planned and implemented in accordance with the Essential Areas and Policies of the Accreditation Council for Continuing Medical Education (ACCME) through the joint sponsorship of the University of Virginia School of Medicine and Elsevier. The University of Virginia School of Medicine is accredited by the ACCME to provide continuing medical education for physicians.

The University of Virginia School of Medicine designates this educational activity for a maximum of 15 *AMA PRA Category 1 Credits*™ for each issue, 60 credits per year. Physicians should only claim credit commensurate with the extent of their participation in the activity.

The American Medical Association has determined that physicians not licensed in the US who participate in this CME activity are eligible for a maximum of 15 *AMA PRA Category 1 Credits*™ for each issue, 60 credits per year.

Category 1 credit can be earned by reading the text material, taking the CME examination online at http://www.theclinics.com/home/cme, and completing the evaluation. After taking the test, you will be required to review any and all incorrect answers. Following completion of the test and evaluation, your credit will be awarded and you may print your certificate.

FACULTY DISCLOSURE/CONFLICT OF INTEREST

The University of Virginia School of Medicine, as an ACCME accredited provider, endorses and strives to comply with the Accreditation Council for Continuing Medical Education (ACCME) Standards of Commercial Support, Commonwealth of Virginia statutes, University of Virginia policies and procedures, and associated federal and private regulations and guidelines on the need for disclosure and monitoring of proprietary and financial interests that may affect the scientific integrity and balance of content delivered in continuing medical education activities under our auspices.

The University of Virginia School of Medicine requires that all CME activities accredited through this institution be developed independently and be scientifically rigorous, balanced and objective in the presentation/discussion of its content, theories and practices.

All authors/editors participating in an accredited CME activity are expected to disclose to the readers relevant financial relationships with commercial entities occurring within the past 12 months (such as grants or research support, employee, consultant, stock holder, member of speakers bureau, etc.). The University of Virginia School of Medicine will employ appropriate mechanisms to resolve potential conflicts of interest to maintain the standards of fair and balanced education to the reader. Questions about specific strategies can be directed to the Office of Continuing Medical Education, University of Virginia School of Medicine, Charlottesville, Virginia.

The faculty and staff of the University of Virginia Office of Continuing Medical Education have no financial affiliations to disclose.

The authors/editors listed below have identified no professional or financial affiliations for themselves or their spouse/partner:
Shayna Flash, PA-C, MPH; Carla Holloway (Acquisitions Editor); William Irvin, MD (Test Author); Douglas W. Laube, MD, MEd (Guest Editor); Benjamin C. Marcus, MD; Marco A. Pelosi, II, MD, FICS; and Marco A. Pelosi, III, MD, FICS.

The authors/editors listed below identified the following professional or financial affiliations for themselves or their spouse/partner:
Alastair Carruthers, MD is an industry funded research-investigator, a consultant, and is on the Advisory Committee/Board for Allergan Inc and MERZ GmbH.
Jean Carruthers, MD is a consultant for Allergan, Merz GmbH, Merz Aesthetics USA, and Lumenis Medical Lasers.
Jay M. Kulkin, MD, MBA is on the Speakers' Bureau for Cynosure, and owns stock in Cynosure.
William F. Rayburn, MD, MBA (Consulting Editor) is an industry funded research/investigator and a consultant for Cytokine PharmaSciences.
Barbara Soltes, MD receives research support from Boeringer Ingelheim, Biosante, Bayer Pharmaceuticals, and Neurocrine; and is on the Speakers' Bureau for TEVA Pharmaceuticals, Lilly Pharmaceuticals, and Warner Chilcott.

Disclosure of Discussion of non-FDA approved uses for pharmaceutical products and/or medical devices:
The University of Virginia School of Medicine, as an ACCME provider, requires that all faculty presenters identify and disclose any off-label uses for pharmaceutical and medical device products. The University of Virginia School of Medicine recommends that each physician fully review all the available data on new products or procedures prior to clinical use.

TO ENROLL

To enroll in the Obstetrics and Gynecology Clinics of North America Continuing Medical Education program, call customer service at 1-800-654-2452 or visit us online at www.theclinics.com/home/cme. The CME program is available to subscribers for an additional fee of $180.00.

Contributors

CONSULTING EDITOR

WILLIAM F. RAYBURN, MD, MBA
Randolph Seligman Professor and Chair, Department of Obstetrics and Gynecology;
Chief of Staff, University Hospital, University of New Mexico Health Science Center,
Albuquerque, New Mexico

GUEST EDITOR

DOUGLAS W. LAUBE, MD, MEd
Professor, Department of Obstetrics and Gynecology, University of Wisconsin School
of Medicine and Public Health, Madison, Wisconsin

AUTHORS

DIANE BERSON, MD
Assistant Clinical Professor, Department of Dermatology, Weill Cornell Medical College
of Cornell University, New York, New York

ALASTAIR CARRUTHERS, MD
Clinical Professor, Department of Dermatology and Skin Science, University of British
Columbia, Vancoucer, British Columbia, Canada

JEAN CARRUTHERS, MD
Clinical Professor, Department of Ophthalmology and Visual Sciences, University
of British Columbia, Vancouver, British Columbia, Canada

SHAYNA FLASH, PA-C, MPH
Physician Assistant, Women's Institute for Health PC, Atlanta, Georgia

JAY M. KULKIN, MD, MBA, FACOG
President, Women's Institute for Health PC, Atlanta, Georgia

MARY P. LUPO, MD
Clinical Professor, Department of Dermatology, Tulane Medical School; Lupo Center
for Aesthetic and General Dermatology, New Orleans, Louisiana

BENJAMIN C. MARCUS, MD
Director of Facial Plastic Surgery, Division of Otolaryngology, Department of Surgery,
University of Wisconsin, Madison, Wisconsin

MARCO A. PELOSI II, MD, FACOG, FACS, FICS
Founder, International Society of Cosmetogynecology; Director, Pelosi Medical Center,
Bayonne, New Jersey

MARCO A. PELOSI III, MD, FACOG, FACS, FICS
Chairman, Obstetrics and Gynecology, International College of Surgeons-United States
Section; Founder, International Society of Cosmetogynecology; Director, Pelosi Medical
Center, Bayonne, New Jersey

ANETTA E. RESZKO, MD, PhD
Department of Dermatology, Weill Cornell Medical College of Cornell University,
New York, New York

BARBARA SOLTES, MD
Associate Professor, Department of Obstetrics/Gynecology, Division of Reproductive
Endocrinology, Rush-Presbyterian-St Luke's Medical Center, Chicago, Illinois

Contents

> Liposuction is the most common cosmetic surgical procedure worldwide. It provides effective contouring of the torso, extremities, and submental areas in properly selected patients. Tumescent liposuction, a local anesthesia technique, and superwet liposuction, a systemic anesthesia technique, are the most common methods. The safety profile of both methods is excellent, but local anesthesia avoids the specific risks associated with general anesthesia. The most common complications of liposuction are contour irregularities and transient bruising. No technology seems to provide superior results over conventional methods.

> Adding volume to the aging face is a notion that has come into vogue as of late but is, however, not a new idea. With the advent of miro-liposuction techniques, there is renewed interest in the use of aspirated fat. Commercial fillers have a valuable place in the cosmetic surgeon's armamentarium and offer immediate volume correction with a more modest financial commitment. Nevertheless, the standardization of fat grafting techniques marks an exciting shift in facial aesthetics with the ability to correct all aspects of the aging face with safe, natural, and lasting results.

> Breast augmentation is the most commonly performed cosmetic procedure among American women. Saline implants, silicone implants, and autologous fat injections are the most common options. The inframammary, periareolar, and axillary routes with or without endoscopy are the most common routes of implantation. The subpectoral dual-plane and the subglandular plane are the most common pockets. The most common complications are capsular contracture for implants and volume loss for injected fat. Breast augmentation does not appear to increase breast cancer risk or survival rates.

> Cosmeceuticals are topically applied products that are more than merely cosmetic, yet are not true drugs that have undergone rigorous placebo controlled studies for safety and efficacy. There are many review articles that outline the theoretical biologic and clinical actions of these cosmeceuticals and their various ingredients. This article reviews how to incorporate various cosmeceuticals into the treatment regime of patients, depending on the diagnosis and therapies chosen. The practical application of when, why, and on whom to use different products will enable dermatologists to improve the methodology of product selection and, ultimately, improve patient's clinical results.

Since its initial approval by the US Food and Drug Administration (FDA) 20 years ago for the treatment of strabismus, hemifacial spasm, and blepharospasm in adults, botulinum toxin (BTX) has become one of the most frequently requested products in cosmetic rejuvenation around the world. After years of clinical success and consistent safety in the upper face, the use of BTX has expanded and evolved to include increasingly complicated indications. In the hands of adept injectors, the focus has shifted from the treatment of individual dynamic rhytides to shaping, contouring, and sculpting, alone or in combination with other cosmetic procedures, to enhance the aesthetic appearance of the face. Although recent reports have questioned the safety of BTX, 25 years of therapeutic and over 20 years of cosmetic use has demonstrated an impressive record of safety and efficacy when used appropriately by experienced injectors.

FORTHCOMING ISSUES

March 2011
Practical Approaches to Controversies in Obstetrical Care
George Saade, MD and
Sean Blackwell, MD, *Guest Editors*

June 2011
Advances in Hysteroscopy
Michael Traynor, MD, MPH, *Guest Editor*

September 2011
Perimenopause
Nanette Santoro, MD, *Guest Editor*

RECENT ISSUES

September 2010
Prevention and Management of Complications from Gynecologic Surgery
Howard T. Sharp, MD, *Guest Editor*

June 2010
Update on Medical Disorders in Pregnancy
Judith U. Hibbard, MD, *Guest Editor*

March 2010
Genetic Screening and Counseling
Anthony R. Gregg, MD and
Joe Leigh Simpson, MD, *Guest Editors*

THE CLINICS ARE NOW AVAILABLE ONLINE!

Access your subscription at:
www.theclinics.com

Foreword

Cosmetic Procedures in Gynecology

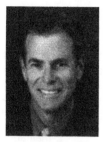

William F. Rayburn, MD, MBA
Consulting Editor

I have been eager to review this issue dealing with cosmetic procedures in gynecology by guest editor, Douglas Laube, MD, since an obstetrician-gynecologist's practice includes more than reproductive health care. The specialty's broad scope on women's health could include cosmetic procedures in its boundaries, just as it has for primary and preventive care. As cosmetic procedures receive more attention from the media and from patients, there is a corresponding need to determine the obstetrician-gynecologists' role in this evolving field.

"One-stop shopping" for both medical and aesthetic services has much appeal to many but not all women. Aesthetic services provided by the obstetrician-gynecologist fill a need not adequately met by other medical offices, provide safer or more efficacious treatments than those available in nonmedical settings, or may be more convenient. Examples of common cosmetic services that represent extensions of gynecologic care include hair removal and acne treatment to patients with polycystic ovary syndrome.

Procedures covered in this issue are of interest to nearly all of our patients: hair removal, laser vein therapy, liposuction, breast augmentation, and facial rejuvenation. These services require a physician to use ethics in patient counseling and informed consent. It is the responsibility of obstetrician-gynecologists to engage their patients in a dialogue that supports the patients' ability to analyze more effectively and respond to societal or marketing pressures. Our patients look to their obstetrician-gynecologists to distinguish between what is anatomically normal and what is unattainable aesthetic ideal. Caution is needed to avoid unsolicited comments about a need for alteration, when none was either desired or considered previously.

For those physicians offering any cosmetic procedure, the well-being and safety of our patients must be foremost. Obstetrician-gynecologists who offer services typically

Obstet Gynecol Clin N Am 37 (2010) xi–xii
doi:10.1016/j.ogc.2010.10.005
0889-8545/10/$ – see front matter © 2010 Elsevier Inc. All rights reserved.

obgyn.theclinics.com

provided by other specialists need to possess an equivalent level of competence. More evidence-based experience reported in the peer-review medical literature is needed about the safety and outcomes of cosmetic procedures described in this issue.

This issue, prepared by several talented and experienced obstetrician-gynecologists, should activate attention to all providers caring for women who inquire about cosmetic procedures. I hope that information provided herein will aid in the careful consideration of determining a role, if any, for postgraduate education and practice within the realm of gynecology.

William F. Rayburn, MD, MBA
Department of Obstetrics and Gynecology
University of New Mexico School of Medicine
MSC 10 5580; 1 University of New Mexico
Albuquerque, NM 87131-0001, USA

E-mail address:
wrayburn@salud.unm.edu

Preface

Cosmetic Procedures in Gynecology

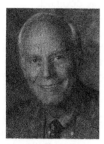

Douglas W. Laube, MD, MEd
Guest Editor

This issue describes cosmetic procedures that can be incorporated into gynecologic practice successfully by additional education and training that is readily available through credible post residency educational programs. While it is recognized that typical post graduate training in obstetrics and gynecology does not provide adequate preparation for the inclusion of cosmetic therapies into safe, quality practice, many obstetricians/gynecologists also recognize that there is not only demand by patients, but also other compelling reasons to consider including these procedures into their scope of practice. In addition to a rapidly growing consumer demand, there are other issues that may affect the obstetrician/gynecologist's decision to learn and provide these treatments, including an ever-expanding unfavorable medical legal climate in providing traditional obstetric and gynecologic services, and the enhanced ability to provide economic sustenance to one's practice.

The scope of practice for the obstetrician/gynecologist has historically included more than reproductive health care, as practitioners have treated such conditions as adolescent pustular acne, hirsuitism, scalp hair loss, and a variety of minor, but unsightly skin lesions. Although the American College of Obstetricians and Gynecologists does not define for the practitioner what her or his scope of practice should be, cosmetic therapy per se is not necessarily excluded provided that the provider has adequate training and experience and functions within an acceptable ethical framework.[1,2]

It would be naïve to assume that financial incentive is not taken into account by the practitioner in considering this type of practice, as consumer demand, industry incentives focused on new devices, and the prospects of a "cash-only" revenue stream have much appeal at a time of diminished revenue through third-party payers. Financial gain

Obstet Gynecol Clin N Am 37 (2010) xiii–xiv
doi:10.1016/j.ogc.2010.10.004
0889-8545/10/$ – see front matter © 2010 Elsevier Inc. All rights reserved.

obgyn.theclinics.com

itself should not condemn the practice of cosmetic therapy; as long as proper ethical boundaries are maintained within the context of patient-generated inquiries into these treatments, therapeutic outcomes are excellent, and patient safety is held paramount.

This issue does not deal with "genital aesthetic surgery," as these procedures are of unproven benefit and remain on the fringe of accepted gynecologic practice.[3] The rigor by which these procedures have been assessed remains suspect, and the training required to attain the required skills has not been openly codified.

I wish to thank the contributors to this issue as respected practitioners within their academic- and community-based institutions. Each has extensive experience in their fields and has written about the subjects presented, while teaching others their skills in a selfless manner. Some are obstetricians/gynecologists by training bringing credibility to the specialty while expanding the boundaries of practice in the health care of women.

Douglas W. Laube, MD, MEd
Department of Obstetrics and Gynecology
University of Wisconsin School of Medicine and Public Health
Madison, WI 53715, USA

E-mail address:
dwlaube@wisc.edu

REFERENCES

1. Code of Professional Ethics of the American College of Obstetricians and Gynecologists. ACOG; 2008.
2. Ethical Decision Making in Obstetrics and Gynecology. ACOG Committee Opinion No. 390. American College of Obstetricians and Gynecologists. Obstet Gynecol 2007;110:1479–87.
3. Surgery and Patient Choice. ACOG Committee Opinion No. 395. American College of Obstetricians and Gynecologists. Obstet Gynecol 2008;111:243–7.

Adding Aesthetics to the OB-GYN Practice

Jay M. Kulkin, MD, MBA*, Shayna Flash, PA-C, MPH

KEYWORDS

- Laser hair removal • Hair reduction • Laser aesthetics
- YAG laser • Alexandrite laser

Laser aesthetic procedures have substantially increased in popularity for both women and men over the past several years. Driven by popular reality makeover television shows and celebrity culture, laser hair removal, spider vein therapy, (Botox) botulinum toxin type A, and other minimally invasive procedures have become an important part of the beauty regimen. As public awareness grows, so does the demand for the safe and effective delivery of these services. In 2008, Americans spent $11.7 billion on aesthetic procedures, representing a 162% increase in the number of aesthetic procedures over 1997.[1] In 2008, 1.3 million laser hair removal procedures were performed, surpassed only by Botox injections.[1] This increase in laser hair removal procedures supports the growing trend of a generation of beauty conscious men and women who view the presence of body hair to be less attractive than smooth skin or people with less hair. A 2006 Harris Interactive survey of 800 women, ages 36 to 69, revealed that on average women would like to look 13 years younger and that they seek aesthetic procedures to accomplish this.[2] With the growing demand for these procedures, many providers of laser services have emerged in the forms of medical spas, laser chains, and laser franchises. Even traditional plastic surgery and dermatology offices have added some of these procedures to accommodate this increase. Because women account for approximately 92% of the aesthetic services market, gynecologists and other primary care providers are offering laser aesthetic procedures to meet their own patient demand.[1] In a managed care environment, aesthetic procedures present an opportunity for clinical practices to venture outside the realm of payment solely by third party and government payers and into the arena of fee for service. These procedures are not based on medical necessity but rather on patient desires. Reimbursement reductions and increasing costs have created an economic crisis, making new profit centers attractive to many practices. As gynecologists develop an expertise in achieving their patients' desired aesthetic results, their practices are faced with caring for a new demographic. Not only do their patients refer

Dr Kulkin is on the Speakers Bureau for Cynosure.
Women's Institute for Health PC, 975 Johnson Ferry Road, Suite 460, Atlanta, GA 30342, USA
* Corresponding author.
E-mail address: jkulkin@wifh.com

Obstet Gynecol Clin N Am 37 (2010) 475–476
doi:10.1016/j.ogc.2010.09.002
0889-8545/10/$ – see front matter © 2010 Elsevier Inc. All rights reserved.

other women to their practice but also patients refer men interested in the same aesthetic results. Although seeing male patients in the gynecology office setting is a new and unique experience, it is well accepted in those practices that have been early adopters of this technology.

PRACTICE MANAGEMENT ISSUES—ADDING AESTHETICS

There are several issues that must be considered when contemplating the addition of laser aesthetics to a gynecology practice. Although medical patients have grown accustomed to waiting for a doctor appointment and having their fee paid by insurance benefits, aesthetic patients are paying their bills out of their personal funds. As a result, excellent customer service must be considered as part of the experience. Patients expect timely appointments, a caring staff, and quality information for the procedures offered. This mandates staff training and dedicating some staff members to care for aesthetic patients. The laser treatment room must have appropriate signage indicating a laser is in use, so that anyone who enters has appropriate eye protection. Each treatment room must have adequate cooling because the lasers themselves produce a fair amount of heat. Individual cooling units in examination rooms are not typical and may need to be refitted. Patients must be able to remove makeup and lotions from treatment areas and razors should be available to remove excess hair before laser treatment. Aftercare products, including *Aloe vera* gel, sunscreen, and deodorant, should be available as well.

MARKETING

Aesthetic procedures are quite different from the typical medical procedures in gynecology. These are procedures patients have seen on television and in the media. Pamphlets discussing the aesthetic procedures offered should be readily available in the office. Practice Web sites should dedicate portions to aesthetic procedures. These procedures should be included in all communications from a practice. As a rule, patients are having these procedures done elsewhere and it is important that they know gynecologists offer them. Prices for services must be readily available and be competitive in the local market.

REFERENCES

1. American Society for Aesthetic Plastic Surgery 2008 data. Available at: ASPS.org 2008. Accessed April 15, 2010.
2. ASPS/Harris Interactive. Perception of the injection. American women's perception of cosmetic facial injectables. ASPS/Harris Interactive; 2006.

Laser Hair Removal

Jay M. Kulkin, MD, MBA*, Shayna Flash, PA-C, MPH

KEYWORDS

• Laser hair removal • Hair reduction • Laser aesthetics
• YAG laser • Alexandrite laser

LASER HAIR REMOVAL: HOW IT WORKS

Since the 1960s physicians have been using lasers for the removal of unwanted hair. A laser (Light Amplification through Stimulated Emission of Radiation) beam is a single wavelength of light, which may be absorbed differently by different targets or chromophores. Gynecologists have experience with many lasers, including, but not limited to, the carbon-dioxide and Nd:YAG lasers. They have used lasers in the treatment of endometriosis and human papillomavirus infection and to perform endometrial ablations. As water is the chromophore for carbon-dioxide laser therapy for human papillomavirus infection, laser hair removal is based on the absorption of laser energy by melanin, the pigment in the hair follicles. Just as the energy from the sun is absorbed by the black color in clothing, producing a large amount of heat, when applied to the skin surface, laser energy is absorbed by the melanin in the hair follicle, creating a significant amount of heat. This heat damages or destroys the hair follicle. Laymen refer to this process as laser hair removal; however, the process is more accurately referred to as laser hair reduction. It is considered a reduction because there is a decrease in the number of hair follicles before and after laser energy application.[1] Of course, the challenge in performing this procedure is to destroy unwanted hair while not damaging the surrounding skin. After the Food and Drug Administration approved the first device for permanent hair reduction, numerous technological advances have allowed clinicians to perform this procedure on all skin types, with excellent results, minimal side effects, and minimal complications.

OFFICE CONSULTATION: IS THE PATIENT A CANDIDATE FOR LASER HAIR REMOVAL?
The Medical History

It is important to understand why patients seek laser hair reduction. Many patients simply have unwanted hair they choose to remove, whereas others experience excessive hair growth due to medical conditions. In the bikini, neck, and axillary areas, many people suffer from ingrown hairs and folliculitis, whereas some have suffered from

J.M.K. is on the Speakers Bureau for Cynosure.
Women's Institute for Health PC, 975 Johnson Ferry Road, Suite 460, Atlanta, GA 30342, USA
* Corresponding author.
E-mail address: jkulkin@wifh.com

Obstet Gynecol Clin N Am 37 (2010) 477–487
doi:10.1016/j.ogc.2010.10.001
0889-8545/10/$ – see front matter © 2010 Elsevier Inc. All rights reserved.

follicular abscesses requiring drainage. These patients seek laser hair removal to prevent recurrences. Laser hair removal prevents ingrown hairs from occurring, making these people more comfortable while achieving a cosmetically favorable result. For female patients with polycystic ovary syndrome or other androgen syndrome, unwanted facial hair presents both physical and emotional issues.[2] Because of male pattern facial hair growth, many of these women suffer from depression and low self-esteem and thus benefit greatly from laser therapy.

At the consultation, the absence of contraindications to laser hair reduction is established. Medical issues that make a candidate unsuitable for laser hair removal include an open bacterial or viral wound in the area to be treated, use of isotretinoin (Accutane) in the previous 6 months, and any history of having received a gold injection for arthritis.[1] Each issue results in skin discoloration, which may be permanent. Although studies on the duration one should be off isotretinoin to avoid skin discoloration are conflicting, a conservative approach to the elective removal of unwanted hair is warranted. Patients with a history of oral or genital herpes are treated prophylactically with an antiviral agent, with the treatment beginning the day before laser therapy and continuing for 1 day after therapy, because laser therapy may reduce the threshold for developing an outbreak.[1] Those patients with an active lesion must schedule their appointment after complete resolution of the outbreak.

The authors choose not to treat pregnant women for purely medicolegal reasons, although no studies have been conducted to indicate any adverse effects. Patients with seizure disorders in whom the seizures are triggered by strobe lights may be treated with the laser; however, use of stainless steel goggles that preclude visualization of the pulsing light is indicated as a precaution. It is important to be aware of areas with permanent makeup or tattoos so that these pigmented areas may be avoided to eliminate the risk of laser absorption. Other medications including light-sensitizing antibiotics or herbal remedies have not presented an issue in the authors' experience of more than 100,000 procedures. A history of skin cancer of any type is not a contraindication for performing laser hair reduction, although a good laser technique mandates avoiding laser contact with pigmented lesions. Laser alters the cellular architecture of these lesions, making pathologic diagnosis more challenging at a later date.

Patients with white or gray hair are not good candidates for laser hair removal because of the lack of melanin in the hair. In addition, some patients with red hair do not respond, whereas others do. This difference in response depends on the amount of melanin in the follicle and can be assessed by test pulses to measure the clearance or the hair's reaction to the laser. Should the hair demonstrate no reaction to a test pulse, the prognosis for an excellent outcome is poor.

At the consultation, the patient's skin type should be established based on the Fitzpatrick scale (**Box 1**). Although this scale has been the standard when choosing a laser appropriate for any given patient, it is important to note that skin color varies naturally on different body parts and after sun exposure and artificial tanning. Light skin types (I–III) may typically be treated with short-wavelength lasers (alexandrite, 755 nm or diode, 800 nm), whereas dark skin types (IV–VI) are safely treated with long-wavelength lasers (Nd:YAG, 1064 nm).

Setting Expectations for Results

Laser hair removal is requested by a wide range of patients representing all skin types. Because first-generation lasers cause burns in ethnic skin, many patients with dark skin types have "heard" they are not candidates for laser therapy. Recent advances in laser technology make this procedure safe for all skin types. It is important from the outset that the patient is counseled to have reasonable expectations about the

> **Box 1**
> **Fitzpatrick skin types**
>
> Type I: Always burns, never tans, and light-colored hair and eyes
>
> Type II: Usually burns, tans with difficulty, light skin, blue- or light-colored eyes
>
> Type III: Sometimes burns but usually tans, eyes dark in color, slightly colored skin (eg, Northern Mediterranean or Asian)
>
> Type IV: Rarely burns, tans easily, dark-colored eyes, definite darkening of skin color
>
> Type V: Very rarely burns, dark-colored hair and eyes (eg, Southern Indian, Spanish, Spanish-African American)
>
> Type VI: Very dark skin color, dark coarse hair, dark eyes (eg, African)

procedure. After a series of 6 to 8 sessions, spaced at 6-week intervals, an 80% reduction of hair is a reasonable expectation.[3] It is important to state candidly that a 100% reduction of hair is extremely rare, although many advertisements guarantee such claims. Some follicles are simply less sensitive to laser therapy, whereas others may be resistant. As a result, those follicles that are damaged, but not destroyed, produce finer slower-growing hair after treatment. Although many patients report shaving daily before laser therapy, they are expected to shave the treated area approximately once a week after treatment. The definition of shaving, however, is different after laser therapy. Patients discover that they have very few hairs in random places on each body part, which makes shaving much quicker and easier than before laser treatment. In addition, razor burn and ingrown hairs are eliminated. The unique characteristics of each body part and its response to laser therapy are discussed later. Some patients may be more fortunate and find their shaving needs reduced to once each month. The authors have been unable to predict which patients will shave weekly and which will shave monthly. Because black hair contains more melanin than brown hair and thick hair contains more melanin than fine hair, a thick, coarse, dark hair is expected to absorb more laser energy, resulting in maximum reduction. This fact should be explained to patients, so that patients with very fine hair may expect a slightly lesser result than another patient who may have thick dark hair.

All body parts, except the eyebrows, may be treated with laser. Retinal injury, caused by the absorption of scattered laser energy during eyebrow hair removal, may result in permanent eye damage. Therefore, eyebrow treatment is contraindicated. The most common areas treated are the face or parts of the face, such as the chin, lip, or sideburns; neck; chest; abdomen; bikini area; back; arms; legs; and buttocks. Because many women have had temporary hair removal techniques, such as waxing, before seeking laser therapy, they frequently request a "Brazilian bikini" style laser treatment in which all or almost all of the hair is removed. Treating the perianal, perirectal, clitoral, and labial areas requires unique laser requirements, which are discussed later.

Consents and Photographs

Patients should be informed of the benefits and risks of laser hair reduction, and a signed document should be included in the medical record. The consent should not offer guarantees and should describe pertinent side effects. If possible, photographs of areas to be treated should be taken before the first session. Some patients may feel uncomfortable with photographs, and their wishes must be respected. In reality, patient satisfaction is the most important indicator for a cosmetically pleasing result. Should a patient express dissatisfaction with the results of a treatment series, consultation with the provider will determine whether additional treatments will be of benefit. Before and after photographs are particularly useful in this situation because experience has shown that patients forget their "before appearance."

WHAT TO EXPECT FROM EACH SESSION—EFFECTS AND SIDE EFFECTS

Patients are advised to shave the area to be treated on the day of or 1 day before their treatment session. Many women not accustomed to shaving their face may feel uncomfortable with shaving and are advised to come to the office without shaving. Clinicians may use disposable razors to gently shave hair off the skin surface to avoid heat absorption by the hair, which may cause crusting. To avoid topical reactions or complications, patients are advised to remove all makeup and lotion thoroughly before laser treatment. These substances often contain pigments that absorb laser energy, resulting in blister development. In the bikini area, patients are advised to shave the area as they would like it to look when laser therapy is complete, and those shaven areas are treated at each session.

The initial session begins by choosing the appropriate laser settings (fluence = power, pulse width = duration of each laser pulse) and cooler settings for the patient's skin and hair types. Clinicians should be sensitive to the apprehension felt by many patients having their first laser treatment. Appropriate eye protection for the wavelength used are worn by all individuals in the treatment room. Working slowly during the first session and explaining everything that transpires can relieve the patient's anxiety. The laser spot size is chosen based on the size of the area to be treated. During a treatment session, the entire surface of the treated area is covered with laser pulses in an orderly fashion of rows, with minimal overlap of each pulse and each row. The laser beam is moved constantly to avoid double pulsing over the same spot producing excess heat development and burns. Patients experience a rubber band–snapping sensation on the skin, which for some patients is uncomfortable. Approximately 25% of patients require a topical anesthetic. Although facial hair reduction rarely requires a topical anesthetic, the back, chest, and abdomen of men often do. Women find axilla treatments painful; however, the procedure requires approximately 3 minutes to perform and as a result is well tolerated. Although discomfort is common while the laser is pulsing, there is complete pain resolution immediately on stopping the laser pulse. Patients leave the office pain free and may return to their regular activity immediately.

Patients do not experience immediate hair reduction but rather see a regrowth of hair beginning within 2 days of each procedure. Approximately 2 to 3 weeks after each session, patients notice hair reduction as well as a reduction of ingrown hair and razor burn. Although marked reduction of up to 50% may be seen after the first session, it should not be perceived as permanent because 6 to 10 weeks later regrowth will become evident. Patients should be counseled to expect long-term permanent reduction after a series of treatments and should not be misled by spurious excessive reduction after the first session.

Between sessions patients may shave as much as they prefer; however, plucking, waxing, threading, tweezing, and use of depilatory agents should be avoided. It is thought that any of these methods may stimulate the follicles to repair the damage inflicted by the laser beam and decrease the amount of total hair reduction. It is preferable that follicles remain at rest so that further damage may be inflicted at each subsequent session.

Lasers for hair reduction have various types of cooling systems to protect the skin from burning. Some use contact cooling, whereas others use air or chemical cooling. The cooling systems can get the skin to temperatures as low as $-4°C$. As a result, mild skin erythema is seen after almost all sessions. As laser energy increases the temperatures in the hair follicles, small hivelike skin eruptions, follicular edema, are seen. Follicular edema is a desired end point of each session, indicating successful energy delivery to the follicle. Women typically experience rapid resolution of follicular edema in minutes, whereas men may experience persistence, with the follicular edema lasting from hours to several days. Although follicular edema is typically asymptomatic, occasionally pruritus can occur and responds well to aloe vera lotion or hydrocortisone lotion, 1%.[4]

Side Effects

Adverse effects from laser hair reduction occur in less than 2% of patients. Burns and blisters may occur if laser settings are excessive in any skin type but are extremely rare with a good technique. Dark skin types should be treated with long-wavelength lasers, whereas light skin types are safely treated with the short-wavelength lasers. Persistent erythema may occur and spontaneously resolves over 2 to 3 days, whereas macular rashes requiring treatment with oral steroids are extremely rare. Should a slight excess of laser energy be used for any given skin color, hyperpigmentation may occur.[5] Within minutes to a few hours of a treatment session, patients experience a mild to severe sunburnt feeling on the treated area and the development of brown cigarette burn–like areas. The discomfort resolves in 24 to 48 hours and the circular brown areas typically crust and scab. These areas begin to fade in 3 to 7 days and the crusting peels off. Resultant hypopigmentation may develop in places where the crusting resolved. It may take from weeks to several months for normal repigmentation to be complete. To accelerate the resolution of hyperpigmentation a hydroquinone medication, 4%, may be applied. Avoidance of hyperpigmentation (more common in light Fitzpatrick skin types I–III) requires learning to choose laser settings for each patient's skin color at the time of therapy. Individuals who come for laser therapy after sun exposure have an increased risk of hyperpigmentation if the technician does not adjust the laser settings accordingly. Although permanent hypopigmentation has been reported, it is extremely rare. Careful evaluation of skin color at each visit is extremely important to avoid the inconvenience that hypo- or hyperpigmentation creates for the patient.

Skin Type and Choice of Laser

At the initial session, the skin type of the patient is assessed using the Fitzpatrick skin type scale. As mentioned earlier, light skin types, with minimal amount of melanin in the skin, may be treated with short-wavelength lasers, which have very high melanin absorption rates. The lack of melanin in light skin allows most of the energy to go directly to the hair follicle. Short-wavelength lasers should not be used on dark skin types because the laser energy is absorbed by the skin melanin and results in burns or blisters. The first ruby red lasers used years ago for hair reduction had an extremely high absorption rate by melanin. When used in dark skin types, ruby red lasers resulted in many burns, which made people of color think they were not candidates for laser therapy. Recent development of the Nd:YAG laser (1064 nm) has resulted in the ability to treat dark skin types safely. These lasers pass through the skin pigment and target the melanin in the hair follicle. This phenomena of selective thermolysis is the process that has allowed clinicians to perform more than 40,000 procedures on dark skin type patients, without even one burn.[6]

In this regard, it is equally important to further assess the skin color carefully in different portions of one anatomic area. In the vaginal area, when treating the bikini area, one must recognize that the labia often contain more melanin than the suprapubic region. Therefore, the suprapubic region may be treated with a short-wavelength laser, whereas the labia may require low-power settings or a long-wavelength Nd:YAG laser to protect the skin. Similarly, while driving, the left arm is subjected to more sun exposure than the right arm. Thus, more tanning may be noticed on the left arm than the right, and care must be taken with setting the laser.

Caveats for Various Body Parts

This section is a guide to unique issues related to many of the areas treated for laser hair reduction. This section can be used as a guide to assist in treating the various areas. All treatment times are approximate.

Facial hair in women

The face is the most common area that patients request to be treated. Women have been using temporary hair removal techniques such as waxing, plucking, threading, and electrolysis for many years. Although permanent hair reduction is accomplished on all body areas, facial follicles seem to continue to grow more readily than follicles on the remainder of the body. Hence, patients are counseled to undergo touch-up sessions approximately 2 to 3 times each year after a series of treatment sessions. Androgen syndromes such as polycystic ovary syndrome, insulin resistance, and androgen hypersensitivity syndromes are associated with slightly less hair reduction and more frequent touch-up sessions **(Fig. 1)**. These patients, do however, find laser hair reduction to be the most effective method. In addition, women with very fine hair and type 1 skin may present a challenge because of the minimal melanin content of their hair. Ethnic women often present with pseudofolliculitis barbae (PFB) **(Fig. 2)**, a condition of ingrown hair, hair bumps, and inflammatory pigmentation on the face and neck.[7] Laser therapy is extremely effective for these women, and they also require touch-up therapy to maintain their excellent results. Ethnic women from areas of South Asia, Eastern Europe, and the Middle East present a unique challenge because they respond well to laser therapy for the lip and chin but show suboptimal responses to the cheek and forehead. As clinicians gain more experience with hair reduction techniques, these nuances become more familiar. The chin, in general, responds

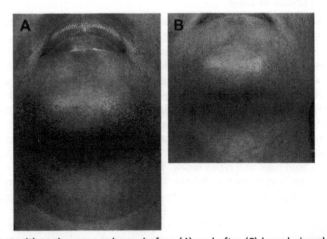

Fig. 1. Patient with androgen syndrome before (A) and after (B) laser hair reduction.

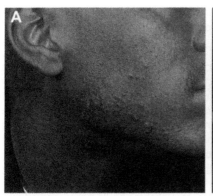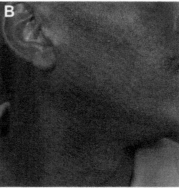

Fig. 2. Patient with PFB before (*A*) and after (*B*) laser hair reduction.

well to laser hair removal therapy, whereas the lip is a bit more challenging because of the presence of fine hair (treatment time, 15 minutes).

Facial hair in men
Men's beards present a unique challenge for laser therapy. The follicle seems to be the most sensitive to testosterone, yet the results are excellent. Because the hair is so coarse and dense, large amounts of laser energy are absorbed creating large amounts of heat, which is uncomfortable. Hence, a low-power setting should be chosen to establish adequate visible clearance of hair, with each laser pulse delivered at 1 pulse per second. As hair is reduced over subsequent sessions, high-power settings and higher rates of delivery may be chosen. Men should be counseled that they still require shaving but less frequently. Typically, after laser therapy, men shave approximately twice weekly; however, the shaving experience is much easier as the remaining hair is finer. Razor burn is markedly reduced or absent, but men are expected to undergo touch-up sessions 2 to 3 times yearly. PFB is also common in men with dark skin types and responds as well as in women (treatment time, 15 minutes).

Neck hair in women and men
Although patients with unwanted neck hair often have facial hair as well, the neck is often treated separately. PFB may present solely on the neck as can razor burn in light skin types. Both men and women may expect excellent results, with touch-ups done at 4- to 5-month intervals to maintain the progress (treatment time, 15 minutes).

Chest and breast hair in women
Chest hair in women (between or above the breast) responds well to laser therapy. Chest hair is often associated with hormonal issues or ethnic predispositions. All parts of the chest and breast may be safely treated. The areola does not contain melanin and may be treated with short-wavelength lasers, without an increased risk of hyper-pigmentation or burns (treatment time, 15 minutes).

Chest and abdomen hair in men
These 2 areas are coarse, dense, and very sensitive, often requiring the use of topical anesthetics. The chest skin color is often significantly lighter than the abdominal skin. Men often request that these 2 areas and the back be treated together. The issue discussed later relative to avoiding large volumes of topical anesthetic applications applies here. Treating the chest and abdomen a day before treating the back is

prudent. Slow repetition rates are warranted until significant reduction is accomplished, at which time faster rates may be used (treatment time, 30–45 minutes).

Bikini area hair in women
This area responds well to treatment and requires a topical anesthetic approximately 25% of the time. All areas may be treated, including the periclitoral and perianal areas. Care must be taken in women with light skin types because the area at the top of the thigh and medial thigh may have been subjected to sun exposure when the patient wears a swimsuit. These sun-exposed areas may require less energy to reduce the risk of hyperpigmentation. At times, the labial skin and perianal areas may be significantly darker than the skin on the pubis. This disparity may allow a short-wavelength laser to be used on the light areas and a long-wavelength laser on the dark areas. In patients with light skin types, use of long-wavelength lasers, which have lower melanin absorption rates, may result in less hair reduction than short-wavelength lasers. Patients should be counseled accordingly and are typically comfortable with this setting. The labia and perirectal areas may be very sensitive to laser energy (treatment time, approximately 15 minutes).

Bikini area hair in men
Rules that are similar to treating the women's bikini area apply to treating the men's bikini area. Again, dark skin areas must be treated with long-wavelength lasers and areas around the testicles may be sensitive, requiring a topical anesthetic (treatment time, 15 minutes).

Leg hair in women and men
Response is good in these areas. The lower leg tends to have thick dense hair and as a result is more sensitive. Bony areas including the toes, feet, shin, and ankle tend to be most sensitive. The medial thigh is often the site of dense thick hair that gets well reduced. The thigh often has very fine hair in light skin types, which may not respond well (treatment time, approximately 1 hour).

Underarm hair in women and men
When treated with laser, the underarm hair follicles tend to respond better than the follicles in other body parts. Shaving less than weekly or even monthly after laser therapy is a typical result for this body part. Even though this area is sensitive, patients tolerate it well because the treatment time is short and the area to be treated is small (treatment time, 5 minutes) (**Fig. 3**).

Back hair in women and men
The back responds well, provided the hair is dark and coarse. Most women present with fine hair and therefore have less reduction than men who present with thick hair. Ethnic women often have bothersome genetic patterns of fine hair, but when counseled to reasonable expectations, these patients are happy with the reduction they achieve. Men with light skin color and fine hair present the same challenge. The shoulders are an area of great resistance often requiring slightly higher fluence. Men typically have significant discomfort in the flank areas, thus requiring a topical anesthetic.

Arm hair in women and men
The arms may have very fine or coarse hair, which of course will dictate the effectiveness of the laser therapy. Conservative settings should be chosen because when hyperpigmentation does occur on the arms, it may lead to a prolonged recovery, up to 1 year.

Hair in the ears and nose
These areas are safely treated using a smaller spot size, typically 3 or 5 mm in diameter. Other than the logistic issue of exposure to areas inside the ear or nasal canal, the

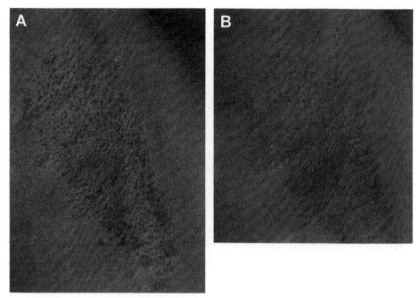

Fig. 3. Patient before (*A*) and after (*B*) underarm hair reduction.

procedure is safe and effective. A tongue depressor assists in exposing these small areas to the laser.

Skin Type and Hair Color Combinations

Patients present with one of the following skin and hair combinations, each with its own set of challenges for the clinician.

Dark hair and light skin

Historically, this combination allows clinicians to use high laser energy and attain maximum absorption by thick dark hair, resulting in maximum reduction. Light skin people should be treated with a short-wavelength laser for maximum effectiveness (**Fig. 4**).

Light hair and light skin

Light hair has substantially less melanin content and requires high laser energy. Compared with patients with dark thick hair, these patients still attain excellent results but must be encouraged to avoid sun exposure. Should these patients become tan, laser settings would have to be reduced to protect the skin and avoid hyperpigmentation, thus attaining suboptimal results.

Dark hair and dark skin

Patients with dark skin types typically have thick, coarse, dark hair. These patients respond well to long-wavelength lasers. In some ethnic patients with dark skin and fine dark hair, a detailed family history often reveals a mixed ethnic background. As a result, the fine hair of these patients may require high fluence levels to attain excellent reduction.

Light hair and dark skin

These patients typically have Fitzpatrick skin types I to III that are tanned or have had sun exposure. This combination provides a significant challenge to attain reduction and requires patients to avoid sun exposure and tanning. The fine light hair, containing

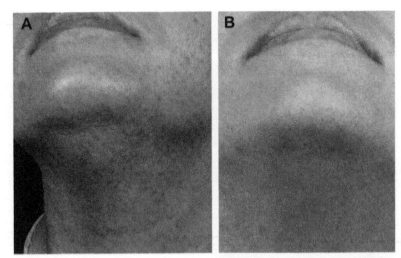

Fig. 4. Before (*A*) and after (*B*) photo of laser hair removal on chin and neck-androgen syndrome.

minimal amount of melanin, requires high fluence settings of the short-wavelength lasers to generate enough heat to damage the hair follicle. These lasers also have such a strong attraction to pigments that the extra melanin content in the tanned skin absorbs the laser energy, resulting in either burns or hyperpigmentation. Although a long-wavelength Nd:YAG (1064 nm) laser may be used safely in these patients, the authors' experience has shown suboptimal results when compared with patients who wait for their tans to subside and are treated with the short-wavelength alexandrite (755 nm) laser.

TOPICAL ANESTHETICS

Although 75% to 80% of patients find laser hair removal procedures tolerable, many people find them too painful. Over-the-counter topical anesthetics and prescription-strength lidocaine creams are typically not potent enough. Compounded products such as Benzocaine, 20% to 40%; lidocaine, 4% to 6%; and tetracaine, 4%, combinations may be applied to the skin 1 hour before the procedure, producing excellent anesthesia. Care must be taken not to cover too much of the body surface to avoid lidocaine toxicity. As a rule, for any given session, application of these potent anesthetics is limited to areas no larger than the legs and bikini area. Occlusion with cellophane should not be done in an attempt to attain superior anesthesia because there have been deaths reported from lidocaine toxicity. Such lethal cases also involved the patients covering large surface areas with the anesthetic.

SUMMARY

Laser hair reduction is a rapidly growing procedure, which may be successfully added to the traditional obstetrics and gynecology practice. Clinicians should seek training in the use of aesthetic lasers and the marketing of their services to achieve optimal outcomes.

REFERENCES

1. Molnar J, Kirman C, Alaiti S, et al. Laser hair removal. Feb 21, 2007. Emedicine from WebMD. Available at: http://www.emedicine.com/plastic/TOPIC438.HTM. Accessed April 15, 2010.
2. Goldberg D, Ahkami R. Evaluation comparing multiple treatments with a 2-msec and 10-msec alexandrite laser for hair removal. Lasers Surg Med 1999;25:223–8.
3. Bashour M, James A, Nassif P, et al. Laser hair removal. Sept 27, 2007. Emedicine from WebMD. Available at: http://www.emedicine.com/ent/TOPIC738.HTM. Accessed April 15, 2010.
4. McDaniel D, Lord J, Ash K, et al. Laser hair removal a review and report on the use of the long-pulsed alexandrite laser for hair reduction of the upper lip, leg, back, and bikini region. Dermatol Surg 1999;25:425–30.
5. DiBernardo B, Perez J, Usal H, et al. Laser hair removal: where are we now? Plast Reconstr Surg 1999;104:247–56.
6. Greidanus T, Honl B, Sperling L, et al. Pseudofolliculitis of the beard. Feb 7, 2007. Emedicine from WebMD. Available at: http://www.emdicine.com/derm/TOPIC354.HTM. Accessed April 15, 2010.
7. Hilton L. Troubles with topicals: FDA warns about numbing creams in wake of two deaths. Dermatology Times April 2007. Available at: http://www.highbeam.com/doc/1P3-1273882591.html. Accessed April 15, 2010.

Intense Pulsed Light Therapy

Barbara Soltes, MD

KEYWORDS

• IPL • Hirsutism • Acne • Phototherapy

The property of light has long been used as a tool for the restoration of health. Hippocrates wrote for decades about the elements of nature as essential components in the balance of sickness and wellness. The healing powers of sunlight became one of the earliest recorded treatments in modern medicine.[1,2] In the early centuries, light treatments were used to correct a wide variety of medical conditions, such as smallpox and tuberculosis.[2] With the advent of the twentieth century, the traditional light treatment was altered and laser emerged as an aesthetic tool. In 1963, Goldman and colleagues[3] first described ruby laser injury to pigmented hair follicles. In the following years, the ruby laser was used to treat other conditions, with little regard for absorption of light energy by various tissues. A historical case reported in 1983 was that of a young boy treated for a vascular nevi with a high-intensity laser, which resulted in severe epidermal damage. In the same year, Anderson and Parrish[4] developed the theory of photothermolysis. This theory was based on pulsed light of a specific wavelength and duration directed at a particular chromophore (melanin, hemoglobin, and water) within the skin layer. The chromophore within a designated tissue could be destroyed selectively, while leaving surrounding tissue unaffected.[4,5] With this concept came an explosion in the number of new light sources in the twenty-first century. These light sources had different wavelengths to accommodate a spectrum of aesthetic procedures with minimal pain.[6–8] In 2008, nearly 75 million aesthetic light procedures were performed, and the number is expected to double because of a growing and demanding young consumer market.

Intense pulsed light (IPL) therapy is an example of an aesthetic light treatment. IPL therapy was initially approved by the US Food and Drug Administration (FDA) in 1998 for photorejuvenation of the pigmented lesions of aging. Shortly thereafter, it was approved for photoepilation and acne photoclearance. IPL therapy has a reputation of being a safe, fast, and effective treatment with a reasonable cost. At present, there are more than 300 registered IPL manufacturers in countries all over the world.[6]

IPL

IPL technology involves parallel xenon flash lamps and capacitors contained within a handheld wand or an articulated arm, which is applied directly to the surface of

Department of Obstetrics and Gynecology, Division of Reproductive Endocrinology, Rush-Presbyterian-St Luke's Medical Center, Chicago, IL 60612, USA
E-mail address: basmd@aol.com

Obstet Gynecol Clin N Am 37 (2010) 489–499
doi:10.1016/j.ogc.2010.09.005
0889-8545/10/$ – see front matter © 2010 Elsevier Inc. All rights reserved.

obgyn.theclinics.com

the skin. Single or multiple pulses of high-intensity light are rapidly discharged to the skin surface. The light travels through the skin at a selected wavelength until it strikes the desired chromophore (**Fig. 1**). The pulsed light is converted to heat energy, which coagulates the desired target, such as a hair bulb or capillary within the dermis of the skin. It does not penetrate deep enough to cause thermal damage to the epidermis. This technique is known as selective photothermolysis. In addition, the IPL wand possesses a filter to remove any ultraviolet (UV) components that lead to UV damage. The pulses of light produced are of very short duration, which minimizes skin discomfort and discoloration.[9]

IPL machinery range from large freestanding units to compact mobile units (**Fig. 2**). The standard properties of an IPL machine provide a wide spectrum of optimal wavelengths, power, and pulse durations. These properties allow for selective photothermolysis for a variety of skin conditions. The usual specifications are as follows:

- Light source delivering a full spectrum of filtered IPL
- Optical adapters or crystal filters with wavelengths of 410 to 1400 nm
- Variable power (energy) range from 26 to 40 J/cm^2
- Variable pulse duration from 5 to 30 milliseconds
- Two pulse modes, single and multidose.

The variability of wavelengths achieved with a simple change of a crystal filter allows for several aesthetic procedures to be done at one visit (**Fig. 3**).[7,10,11]

PATIENT PREPARATION

A complete written medical history is the first requirement of IPL treatment. Absolute contraindications to IPL therapy include seizure disorder, skin cancer, systemic lupus erythematosus, pregnancy, shingles, vitiligo, skin grafts, and open skin lesions. Medications that are associated with photosensitivity (tetracyclines, sulfonylureas, isotretinoin, thiazide diuretics, nonsteroidal antiinflammatory drugs, St John's wort) should not be used while undergoing photo treatments. A relative contraindication to IPL therapy is tanning or sun exposure within 30 days of the procedure. It is important to set expectations and estimate the number of treatments required for a desired

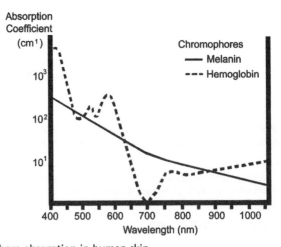

Fig. 1. Chromophore absorption in human skin.

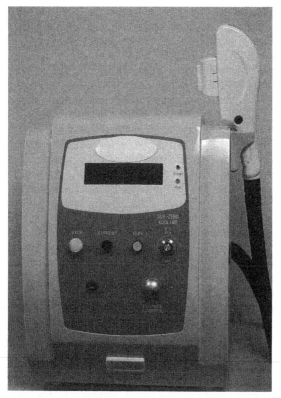

Fig. 2. IPL system.

outcome. Generally, a plan consists of 4 to 6 treatments at monthly intervals. A consent form that explains the potential risks should be obtained before any treatment.[11] The risks include alterations in skin pigmentation and, rarely, scarring at the treatment site.[12]

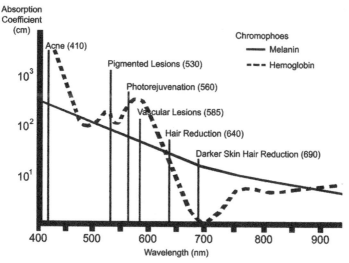

Fig. 3. Wavelength spectrum for clinical indications.

Skin assessment is essential for any phototherapy. The determination of a skin type is made by a self-administered questionnaire. Points are assigned based on genetic composition, reaction to sun exposure, and tanning habits. The final score designates a Fitzpatrick skin type, which correlates well with one of 6 skin types, from very fair (type 1) to very dark (type 6) (**Table 1**). This classification system has been used since 1975 as a proven diagnostic and therapeutic tool in all dermatologic conditions. It was adopted by the FDA for the evaluation of sun protection factor values of current sunscreens.[11,13,14]

Based on the skin type and the photo procedure to be performed, a filter is selected. Filters are wavelength specific; that is, for acne photoclearance, a wavelength of 410 nm is needed, whereas for photoepilation, a wavelength of 640 to 690 nm is selected. Adjustable energy or fluences (26–40 J/cm^2), along with a variable pulse duration (5–30 milliseconds), that is the safest and most efficacious for the desired procedure must be selected. A single pulsed mode is used when higher energy is required, such as photoepilation in a woman with a light skin tone. Multipulsed mode delivers a minipulse, followed by a millisecond delay, and then a final minipulse. The advantage of the multidose mode is that it allows for the epidermis to cool while thermal energy accumulates in a larger chromophore, such as a blood vessel. The skin to be treated must be clean and dry immediately before the photo treatment. No acetone or alcohol should be used. A spot test may be done initially to determine the most effective power level for a particular skin type and condition.[11,14,15] Protective eyewear should be used to avoid retinal damage.

The FDA has approved 8 indications for IPL treatments. The 2 indications that would be a suitable addition to any gynecologic practice are photoepilation (hair removal) and acne photoclearance. Only these 2 indications are discussed in further detail. Other indications include photorejuvenation, photoclearance of pigmented lesions and vascular lesions, rosacea, telangiectasias (spider veins), and solar lentigo (brown spots).[7]

Table 1
Fitzpatrick skin classification system

Skin Type	Response to Sun Exposure	Examples	Susceptibility
I	Always sunburn, never tan	White, very fair and freckled Red or blond hair Blue-eyed Celts	Very high
II	Usually sunburn, tan with difficulty	White, fair Red or blond hair Blue, hazel, or green eyes Scandinavians	High
III	Sometimes sunburn, tan gradually	Beige, fair Any hair color Any eye color Very common	Average
IV	Rarely sunburn, tan easily	Brown Dark hair Brown-eyed Mediterranean Caucasian	Low
V	Very rarely sunburn, tan very easily	Dark brown Mideastern Latin American	Very low
VI	Never sunburn, tan very easily	Black	Minimal

APPLICATIONS IN GYNECOLOGY

Hyperandrogenism is a common endocrinopathy in women. Women may present to their gynecologists with distressing signs of androgen excess. Hyperandrogenic states such as acne and hirsutism are encountered and usually treated with a prolonged course of antiandrogenic agents with fair but delayed results. The addition of an adjuvant treatment, such as phototherapy, would lead to a quicker and more permanent solution. It is also a means to supplement revenue in these times of medical reform.

ACNE

Nearly 90% of adolescents and 20% of all adult women experience acne at some point in their lives. Many women complain of hormonal acne, which correlates to hormonal changes in their menstrual cycle. Traditional therapies include topical creams or lotions, which cause redness and irritation of the skin. Oral antibiotics are also used, but recent studies indicate an associated 40% resistance rate. In the United States, an estimated $1.4 billion is spent yearly on these treatments with less-than-satisfactory results.[8,15]

Sunlight has long been known to improve acne. However, the visible violet light present in sunlight also has long-term skin damaging effects that preclude it as a reasonable treatment option. IPL therapy uses the same band of wavelength (420 nm) along with filtering of UV rays to safely eradicate the sebum and bacteria in skin pores leading to acne.[16-18]

Skin is composed of an epidermal layer of downward pegs interlocking with dermal papilla of an underlying dermis, both resting on subcutaneous tissue. The outer epidermis is covered by a layer of keratin, which acts as a barrier from outside injury or infection. Within the epidermis are skin pores. Deep within the pores lie the sebaceous glands, which are angled between the hair follicle and epidermis. The glands produce sebum, an oily substance of lipids and wax esters, responsible for skin texture and moisture (**Fig. 4**).[8,14]

The hair follicle is located in both the upper layers of the skin. The depth of the follicle varies at different body sites. The hair follicle undergoes a growth cycle that is influenced by many factors, including hormones. Androgens determine the hair growth rate and the transformation from soft, unpigmented, vellus hair to coarse, pigmented, and permanent terminal hair. In women, the ovaries, the adrenal gland, and the

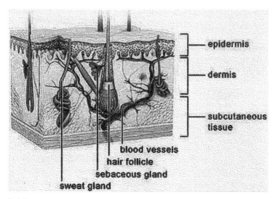

Fig. 4. Anatomy of skin.

peripheral layer of the skin produce androgens. As hormones change, a hardening of the keratin layer or hyperkeratinization of the skin may occur and result in increased sebum production. This hardening may cause a blockage of the skin pore and hair follicle, creating a closed anaerobic environment.

Propionibacterium acnes bacteria build up and rapidly replicate in an anaerobic environment. These bacteria damage the follicle wall and initiate an inflammatory reaction. In the metabolic processes of *P acnes*, porphyrins are produced. Porphyrins absorb light with a wavelength in the UV range. When porphyrins become chemically active, they induce a photodynamic reaction and subsequently release singlet oxygen or free radicals. The free radicals destroy *P acnes* in the sebaceous glands. Most studies show an 80% improvement with just 3 IPL treatments. IPL therapy has been shown to be far superior to topical agents such as benzoyl peroxide (**Fig. 5**).[17–19]

HIRSUTISM

In the twentieth century, clothes became more revealing and women became focused on the removal of visible body hair. Various types of temporary hair removal are widely used on a seasonal basis, but conditions such as polycystic ovarian disease, in which there is excessive body hair, require a more permanent hair removal solution. Hirsutism is the presence of excessive hair growth in a typical male-pattern distribution. The distribution pattern includes the upper lip, upper arms, forearms, back of neck, chin, central chest, midabdomen, entire pubic region, inner thighs, shoulders, and back.[20]

Hirsutism occurs in 5% to 10% of women of reproductive age and is caused by an excess of androgen. More than 70% of hirsutism in women is caused by polycystic ovarian disease. Although benign, it is an extremely distressing condition because

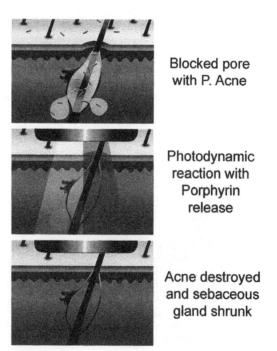

Blocked pore with P. Acne

Photodynamic reaction with Porphyrin release

Acne destroyed and sebaceous gland shrunk

Fig. 5. Acne photoclearance. (*Courtesy of* Sybaritic, Inc, MN; with permission.)

of the excessive hair growth. Antiandrogenic treatments are necessary, but photoepilation is an excellent adjuvant for immediate and more permanent hair removal.[20,21]

A basic understanding of the hair follicle and its growth cycle is essential to the hair removal process. The number of hair follicles is genetically influenced and determined at birth. Women of all ethnicities may have similar estrogen and testosterone levels but differ in the amount of body hair because of the number of hair follicles per unit skin. Scalp hair grows at a rate of 0.4 mm/d or about 6 mm/y. Hair growth and loss is not cyclic or seasonal. A random number of hairs are at various stages of growth and shedding. At the base of the hair follicle is the dermal papilla, which is responsible for the metabolism of nutrients essential for hair growth. It is also the site of androgen receptors. The hair growth response is directly correlated to androgen excess.[22]

There are 3 stages of hair growth: anagen (growth phase), catagen (transitional phase), and telogen (resting phase). Anagen is the active phase of the hair follicle. The stem cells in the bulge are rapidly dividing, and eventually, new hair is formed, which is pushed up the shaft and out the epidermis. Hair grows about 1 cm every 28 days. Scalp hair can stay in this active phase for 2 to 6 years. Hair on the arms or legs has a short anagen phase of 30 to 45 days. Hair loss can occur when the anagen phase is interrupted by medications or various illnesses. Catagen is the transitional phase, and it lasts for about 2 to 3 weeks. About 3% of all hairs are in this phase at any time. During this phase, hair growth stops. Telogen is the resting phase and lasts for about 3 months for scalp hair and longer for arm or leg hair. Nearly 10% to 15% of all hair is found in this phase. About 25 to 100 telogen hairs are shed daily. Excessive shedding during this phase may result a few months after a stressful event, such as childbirth, surgery, or weight loss. After telogen, the hair cycle is complete and anagen restarts. Older hair is pushed out, new hair shafts form, and the cycle repeats itself **(Fig. 6)**.[22,23]

Hair consists of 3 main parts, namely the shaft, bulge, and bulb **(Fig. 7)**. The hair shaft is the visible part of the hair, which has no influence on hair growth, and contains the arrector pili and stem cells, which are important for hair regeneration. The hair bulb is at the base of the follicle where it lies in contact with the dermal papilla. It contains the chromophore melanin. Women with dark hair have greater amounts of melanin and the best results with hair removal using IPL.[22,24,25]

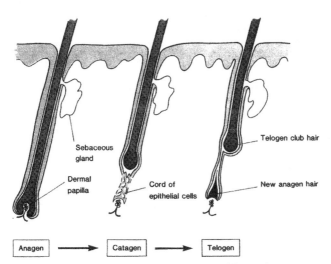

Fig. 6. The hair growth cycle. (*From* Hunter JA, Savin JA, Dahl MV. The structure and function of hair. In: Clinical dermatology. London: Blackwell Scientific; 1989. p. 4–18; with permission.)

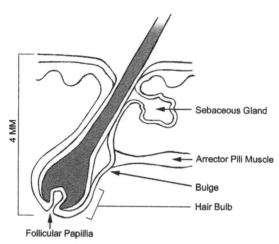

Fig. 7. Anatomy of a hair follicle. (*From* Hunter JA, Savin JA, Dahl MV. The structure and function of hair. In: Clinical dermatology. London: Blackwell Scientific; 1989. p. 4–18; with permission.)

The usual methods of hair removal may be classified into 2 main groups. The first group includes temporary removal, such as depilation (shaving, chemical creams) or epilation (tweezing, waxing). The second group is considered as permanent hair removal, which includes photoepilation (laser or IPL) and electrolysis. For the sake of discussion, photoepilation is the only method addressed in this article.[23,24]

There are many similarities between laser hair removal and IPL therapy. Both procedures are based on selective photothermolysis and target the skin chromophores (melanin, hemoglobin, and water). It is possible to remove 20% to 40% of the hair in the anagen phase in a single treatment. The best results occur in short dark hair on light skin. The results may last for 12 months or longer.[21,24] In spite of the similar actions of these 2 methods, there are some major differences, which are listed in **Table 2**.

Overall, the results of hair removal are the same for both devices, but IPL therapy has gained popularity because of its relatively low cost (about $500 for 6 sessions), minimal discomfort, and the nominal amount of time needed per visit.[21,24–26]

The process of IPL treatment is simple and results in minimal discomfort. IPL is adjusted to a wavelength between 640 and 690 nm in a single pulsed mode, then

Table 2
Comparison of photoepilation techniques

Characteristics	Laser Photoepilation	IPL Photoepilation
Color beam	Monochromatic	Polychromatic
Beam projection	Convergent beam	Divergent beam
Power source	Stimulated emission	Xenon flash lamps
Wavelength	Specific wavelength	Wavelength 400–1400 nm
Filter for wavelength	No filters	Always with a filter
Skin types	I–VI	I–VI
Cost and results	Expensive, slow	Less expensive, fast
Skin contact	No contact with skin	Direct contact with skin
Handpiece (wand)	Small handpiece	Large handpiece

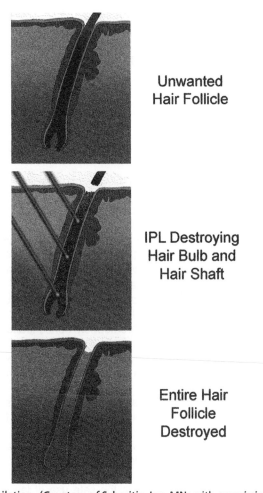

Unwanted
Hair Follicle

IPL Destroying
Hair Bulb and
Hair Shaft

Entire Hair
Follicle
Destroyed

Fig. 8. IPL photo epilation. (*Courtesy of* Sybaritic, Inc, MN; with permission.)

directed to the site of desired hair removal. The duration of pulse frequency correlates positively with the length of the hair to be removed. The longer the hair the greater the pulse frequency. The focused light travels through the skin until it strikes the bulb of the hair. The bulb contains the highest concentration of melanin compared with the rest of the hair shaft. As the light is converted to heat energy, the bulb and most of the hair shaft are coagulated. The intense heat also destroys the hair-producing papilla or the entire hair follicle. To be effective, an adequate amount of heat energy must reach both structures to coagulate them and stop the hair growth. Effective hair reduction is best achieved with hair follicles in the anagen phase. In general, 4-week intervals are required between treatments to yield the best hair removal results (**Fig. 8**).[24–27]

SUMMARY

Light therapy remains an important aspect of medicine. IPL therapy is based on selective photothermolysis, which allows for a rapid treatment with great results and minimal discomfort. It has been proved to be a safe and efficacious phototherapy for a variety of dermatologic and aesthetic conditions. Gynecologists may easily incorporate IPL therapy into their practice with minimal training provided by the manufacturer. It is an acceptable mode of adjuvant therapy for all women who suffer the distressing signs of hyperandrogenism. IPL therapy also carries an added benefit of an additional source of revenue.

REFERENCES

1. Kelly K. The Middle Ages. The history of medicine: the Middle Ages. New York: Infobase Publishing; 2009. p. 1–17.
2. Bettman O. Hippocrates. A pictoral history of medicine. New York: Charles Thomas Publisher; 1979. p. 14–32.
3. Goldman L, Blaney DJ, Kindel DJ, et al. Effect of laser beam on skin. Preliminary report. J Invest Dermatol 1963;40:121–2.
4. Anderson RR, Parrish JA. Selective photothermolysis: precise microsurgery by selective absorption of pulsed radiation. Science 1983;220(4596):524–7.
5. Grossman MC, Dierickx C, Farinelli W. Damage to hair follicles by normal mode ruby laser pulses. J Am Acad Dermatol 1996;35(6):889–94.
6. Tanzi EL, Jason R, Lupton M, et al. Lasers in dermatology: four decades of progress. J Am Acad Dermatol 2003;49:1–31.
7. Tseng SH, Bargo P, Durkin A, et al. Chromophore concentrations, absorption, and scattering properties of human skin in vivo. Opt Express 2009;17:14599–617.
8. Bashkatov AN, Genina EA, Kochubey VI, et al. Optical properties of human skin, subcutaneous and mucous tissues in the wavelength range from 400 to 2000 nm. J Phys D 2005;38:2543–55.
9. Sakamoto FH, Wall T, Avram MM, et al. Lasers and flashlamps in dermatology. In: Fitzpatrick's dermatology in general medicine. New York: McGraw-Hill; 2008. p. 2263–79.
10. Alster TS. Getting started: setting up a laser practice. In: Alster TS, editor. Manual of cutaneous laser techniques. Philadelphia: Lippincott, Williams and Wilkins; 2004. p. 2–4.
11. Wausau WI. Standards of practice for the safe use of lasers in medicine and surgery. American Society for Laser Medicine and Surgery; 1998. p. 1–10.
12. Moreno-Arias GA, Castelo-Branco C, Ferrando J. Side-effects after IPL photodepilation. Dermatol Surg 2002;28(12):1131–4.
13. Sachdeva S. Fitzpatrick skin typing: applications in dermatology. Indian J Dermatol Venereol Leprol 2009;75:93–6.
14. Dover JS, Arndt KA, Dinchart SM, et al. Task force guidelines of care for laser surgery. J Am Acad Dermatol 1999;41:484–95.
15. Dierickx CC, Grossman MC. In: Goldberg DJ, editor. Laser hair removal, lasers and lights. 2005. vol 2. p. 61–6.
16. Papageorgiou P, Katsambas A, Chu A. Phototherapy of blue and red lights in the treatment of acne. Br J Dermatol 2005;142(5):973–8.
17. Ellman M. The effective treatment of acne vulgaris by a high-intensity, narrow band 405–420 nm light source. J Cosmet Laser Ther 2003;2:111–7.
18. Ellman M, Lask G. The role of pulsed light and heat energy in acne clearance. J Invest Dermatol 2004;2:91–5.
19. Cartier H. Use of intense pulsed light in the treatment of scars. J Cosmet Dermatol 2005;4:34–40.
20. Santali A, Shapiro J. Management of hirsutism. Skin Therapy Lett 2009;14(7):1–4.

21. Haedersdal M, Gotzche PC. Laser and photoepilation for unwanted hair growth. Cochrane Database Syst Rev 2006;4:CD0046854.
22. Hunter JA, Savin JA, Dahl MV. The structure and function of hair. In: Clinical dermatology. London: Blackwell Scientific; 1989. p. 4–18.
23. Martin KA, Chang RJ, Ehrmann DA, et al. Evaluation and treatment of hirsutism in premenopausal women: an endocrine society clinical practice guide. Clin Endocrinol Metab 2008;93(4):1105–20.
24. Olsen EA. Methods of hair removal. J Am Acad Dermatol 1999;40:143–55.
25. Liew SH. Unwanted body hair and its removal: a review. Dermatol Surg 1999; 25(6):431–9.
26. Buddhadev RM. Standard guidelines of care: laser and IPL hair reduction. Indian J Dermatol Venereol Leprol 2008;74:S68–74.
27. Amin SP, Goldberg DJ. Clinical comparison of four hair removal lasers and light sources. J Cosmet Laser Ther 2006;8:65–8.

Laser Vein Therapy

Jay M. Kulkin, MD, MBA*, Shayna Flash, PA-C, MPH

KEYWORDS
- Laser vein therapy • Laser aesthetics • Yag laser • Spider
- Veins • Varicose • Laser • Sclerotherapy

As aesthetic procedures gain in popularity, patients are increasingly seeking remedies for the removal of unsightly leg and facial blood vessels. While many gynecologists are introducing laser aesthetic procedures into their practices, there is a need to understand the clinical issue, various treatment modalities, and business decisions to optimize the required investment. This article will introduce the clinician to the very common issue of spider veins, the treatment of which may be accomplished with the same lasers used for laser hair reduction.

The small flat or slightly raised cord-like structures on the legs (**Fig. 1**) are referred to as spider veins.[1] Spider veins may be blue, red, or purple in color and are typically 1 to 2 mm in diameter.[1,2] The larger leg vessels, which are typically wide and bulging, are called varicose veins.

While venous disease affects more than 80 million Americans, the American College of Plastic Surgeons (ASPS) estimates that spider veins occur in approximately 50% of women over the age of 21.[3] While both men and women are subject to spider vein development, typically men do not seek treatment for their spider veins, because their body hair usually covers them up, hence making them less noticeable.[3] Similarly, treatment is sought more frequently by women with lighter skin types, as the contrast between the vessel color and the skin color makes them more noticeable. Spider veins are more common after the age of fifty, and are often due to genetic pre-disposition. One in two people will develop venous varicosities after the age of 50. Pregnancy, obesity, leg injury, prolonged standing, and hormonal therapy, also increase the risk of their development.[1,3]

The venous system brings blood from the extremities to the heart using a series of valves to prevent the reflux of blood back to the extremities.[1] When the valves begin to lose full functionality, blood refluxes back to the extremities, increasing the intravascular pressure.[1] It is this increase in pressure that results in the development of visible spider or varicose veins. Prolonged standing, typically for occupational reasons, may increase back pressure on the valves and increase the risk of this venous issue. In this

Dr Kulkin is on the Speakers Bureau for Cynosure.
Women's Institute for Health PC, 975 Johnson Ferry Road, Suite 460, Atlanta, GA 30342, USA
* Corresponding author.
E-mail address: jkulkin@wifh.com

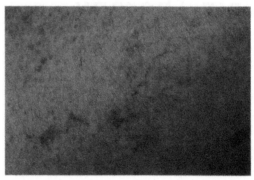

Fig. 1. Spider veins.

regard, pregnancy and obesity, with its resultant increased intra-abdominal pressure on the vena cava, contribute to this venous insufficiency.

Spider veins are not dangerous and do not require medical therapy.[1] More commonly, the treatment of these vessels is done for cosmetic reasons. Women tend to dislike the aesthetic appearance of their leg vessels while wearing shorts, skirts, dresses, and swimsuits. Involvement of the ankles and feet are common as well, further exacerbating the aesthetic issue, especially during warmer weather. Similar to other antiaging procedures like Botox, skin rejuvenation, and facial plastic surgery, spider vein therapy is seen as a way to reverse the signs of aging.

Varicose veins present an entirely different clinical situation. While often asymptomatic, varicose veins may cause throbbing leg pain, worsening with extended periods of ambulation. Leg fatigue, lower extremity skin discoloration, and rashes are also often associated with varicose veins. The pooling of blood in these vessels may result in the development of more serious issues such as superficial or deep vein thrombophlebitis.[1] In addition to thrombophlebitis, life-threatening pulmonary emboli or venous stasis ulcers can occur in more serious cases.[1]

Currently there are few treatment options for spider veins. Historically, one of the more common treatment options has been sclerotherapy, which comes from the Greek word for hardening; it is the injection of sclerosing agents into the vessels.[2,3] This medication causes an inflammatory reaction of the vessel wall, resulting in the development of fibrous tissue, which closes the vessel lumen.[1,2] Due to the limited treatment options, this has been the gold standard for the treatment of both spider veins and varicose veins. Sodium tetradecyl sulfate is the only currently US Food and Drug Administration approved sclerosant. Suffice it to say there are other solutions used as off-label applications. Depending on the volume of vessels to be treated, vessel resolution may be attained in one to three visits. It is common to have bruising last days to weeks, while long lasting or permanent bruising is rare. For this reason, women typically prefer to have their vessels treated during the fall and winter months when their clothing will cover their treated areas.

SIDE EFFECTS AND RISKS

While sclerotherapy is not painful, there may be some discomfort and risk. These risks include deep vein thrombosis, pain, allergy to sclerosing agents, scarring and numbness, edema, and skin ulceration.

Matting of vessels also may occur after sclerotherapy.[3] A matted complex is the development of new spider veins near the treatment areas, creating a complex interconnected network of vessels. When compressed, a rapid, multidirectional filling of the complex is observed. While these may regress spontaneously over several months, they may be extremely difficult to treat.

Contraindications to sclerotherapy include pregnancy, history of deep vein thrombosis, peripheral vascular disease, and systemic diseases such as diabetes or heart disease.

While death from sclerotherapy is extremely rare, isolated cases related to sclerotherapy procedures have been reported.

Patients typically wear medical-grade compression hose for 4 to 6 weeks following the procedure. Ambulation and exercise immediately following the procedure reduce the risk of deep vein thrombosis.

LASER TREATMENT OF SPIDER VEINS

As laser technology has improved, clinicians have been able to use laser therapy to eliminate unsightly spider veins. Many patients choose not to pursue sclerotherapy because of fear of needles and perception of the associated pain, while approaches using lasers are perceived differently. During the 1980s, pulse dye lasers (515–590 nm) and Argon lasers (488 nm and 514 nm) were shown to be effective in the treatment of spider veins.[2,4] In the 1990s, other long wavelength technologies were developed based on the lasers' ability to be absorbed by hemoglobin[4] (**Fig. 2**). Just as melanin is the chromophore for hair reduction lasers, hemoglobin is the chromophore in the treatment of spider veins and varicose veins. The treatment of spider veins with lasers is more complex than laser hair reduction, as numerous wavelengths may be used for

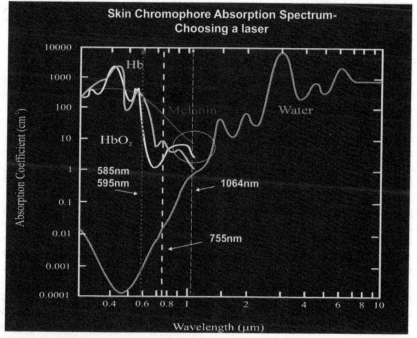

Fig. 2. Hemoglobin absorption curve.

this application. However, wavelengths such as the 1064 NM Nd:YAG, used for the permanent reduction of hair, also may be used for spider vein therapy.

Lasers used to treat spider veins must be absorbed by the hemoglobin in the damaged vessel. As a result of laser energy absorption, heat is generated that must heat the entire endothelium.[4] While this thermal damage coagulates the vessel, one must be careful not to damage the surrounding skin. Cooling devices such as air or contact cooling serve as excellent instruments to accomplish this. Several variables must be considered in the treatment strategy of spider veins.

Contraindications

Unlike sclerotherapy, laser therapy may be used on almost all patients. While pregnant women should not be treated because of the increased intravascular volume and pressure, nursing women may be treated. Similarly, patients with chronic cardiovascular disease and diabetes may be treated. They often find this less invasive therapy quite acceptable without the increased risk of injection complications.

Choosing a Laser

While spider veins may be treated in all skin types, the appropriate laser must first be chosen. In patients with darker skin types, pulse dye lasers, with a strong attraction to melanin, would increase the risk of complications, whereas patients with lighter skin types may be treated with any of the vascular lasers. As a result, in darker skin types, a laser that selectively ignores the skin pigment, such as the Nd:YAG, would be a better choice. Today, the most commonly used lasers for the treatment of spider veins are pulse dye lasers, the Nd:YAG laser, diode lasers, and intense pulse light devices.[4] There are other wavelengths that may be used as well quite effectively. While each wavelength presents a new learning curve to the clinician, the Nd:YAG laser is often already in use in the gynecology practice for laser hair reduction. This allows the clinician to treat the patients most effectively while optimizing the capital investment initially made to offer this service. While the Nd:YAG is effectively absorbed by hemoglobin, there are several laser setting issues that must be understood.

Power or Fluence

The choice of a fluence (power) setting is directly related to the color, size, and depth of the vessel. Spider veins may vary in color on the same patient and on the same extremity. Darker vessels require less energy to treat effectively. As one begins to treat vessels, a visible response will be more easily attained as the color of the vessel gets darker. If the vessels are deeper, more power will be required. A laser spot size directly impacts the depth of energy penetration and therefore should be considered when choosing the power setting for therapy. As the spot size increases so does depth of penetration. While a superficial spider vein is easily treated with a 3 mm spot size, one would consider a larger 5 mm spot for a deeper, larger vessel. As a rule, larger vessels will be located deeper under the skin surface. Slightly larger, blue vessels, referred to as reticular veins, such as those located in the popliteal fossa, may have a slight varicosity to them. Since the reticular veins are located even deeper, they respond nicely to an even larger 7 mm spot size. As a result of these variables, clinicians learn to choose laser settings that combine an appropriate fluence and spot size based on vessel color and location. The last variable to consider is the pulse width, or the time over which the laser energy is delivered. Pulse width may vary from as little as 10 milliseconds to 100 milliseconds. As a rule, the longer the pulse width, the deeper the depth of penetration and the longer the energy is available to impact the vessel. Combining these concepts, it is understood that choosing a large spot size and a long pulse width results in power being delivered deeper and longer. A large reticular vessel would be treated in such a manner, while a superficial spider vein would be treated with a smaller spot size and shorter pulse width. As one gains experience with this treatment modality, more precise settings are chosen repeatedly with more predictable results.

The technique for laser treatment of spider veins is done by placing laser pulses on the vessel and tracing the vessel from one end to the other. Patients are most comfortable wearing shorts, and both legs may be treated during a single session, typically lasting 30 to 40 minutes. While common distributions are a horseshoe pattern" on the lateral thighs and multiple unique areas on the lower legs, patients will each present with their unique problem areas. Patients are treated supine for an anterior vein treatment, with their legs over the end of the treatment table to take advantage of gravity. On occasion, patients may choose to stand, making the treatment area more prevalent for the clinician. The posterior surfaces are treated with patients in a prone or lateral recumbent position. While direction of therapy, from the top or bottom, of the vessel is not critical, cooling, and continuing to move along the vessel, is. One should continue to move the laser to avoid double pulsing on one area; this will help to reduce the risk of blister or burn. A successful pulse will result in a blanching effect as the vessel loses its color and becomes gray. On occasion if a vessel does not blanch a second pass over a vessel may be necessary; this may be done after a short time interval and further cooling to the area. Multiple passes over the same area, however, should be avoided. Treating the ankle area, where the skin is thinner, should be done with approximately 20% to 30% less fluence to avoid complications.

While the procedure is well tolerated, feeling like a rubber band snapping the skin, the treatment of deeper, larger vessels may be quite uncomfortable. Topical anesthetics may be applied safely 1 hour before therapy when necessary. Some patients prefer to take a nonsteroidal anti-inflammatory drug before the procedure. The immediate visible result from successful laser therapy of spider veins is a gray vessel, mild edema directly over the vessel, and erythema (**Fig. 3**). While redness may last a few days, bruising can last days to months. One should avoid using excessively high power, resulting in skin blanching, which may lead to hyperpigmentation or a burn.[4] Patients should be apprised of the rare possibility of permanent bruising. With appropriate laser settings, the incidence of blisters and burns is exceedingly low. Sunscreen should be applied to all areas to reduce the risk of postinflammatory

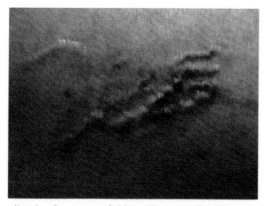

Fig. 3. Results immediately after successful laser therapy of spider veins.

hyperpigmentation.[4] After 2 to 3 months, patients are reassessed to decide if further laser therapy is indicated. Approximately 30% of patients will require an additional laser session.

Once a successful result is attained, patients should be advised that as they age, further spider vein development may occur. There are several things patients can do to prolong the process of development of new spider veins. High heel shoes prevent the flexion of the ankle during walking, thus preventing the calf muscles from effectively pumping blood back to the heart. This creates a venous stasis situation that increases intravascular pressure and the development of more spider veins. Leg elevation may assist venous blood flow and reduce intravascular pressure, thus preventing spider vein development.

Complications

The most common complication related to laser treatment of spider veins is bruising and mild inflammatory hyperpigmentation, which may last from 3 to 6 months. Blisters may occur but are far less common. These are easily treated with topical antibiotics and routine care. Vessel rupture, more common with larger reticular veins, results in immediate swelling. This responds well to ice. Lowering the power settings will prevent this from recurring. As the clinician gains more experience, these issues become less common.

SUMMARY

Laser therapy for the treatment of spider veins is an excellent modality that can easily be incorporated into the contemporary gynecology practice. Clinicians should seek postgraduate medical education sources to learn the applications of these very effective devices.

REFERENCES

1. Weiss M. Varicose veins and spider veins frequently asked questions. The National Women's Health Information Center, US Department of Health and Human Services, Office on Women's Health. Available at: www.hhs.gov, http://www.womenshealth.gov/faq/varicose-spider-veins.cfm. Accessed April 15, 2010.
2. American Academy of Dermatology. Spider vein, varicose vein therapy. Available at: http://www.aad.org/public/publications/pamphlets/cosmetic_spider.html. Accessed April 15, 2010.
3. Encyclopedia of surgery. Sclerotherapy for varicose veins. Available at: http://www.surgeryencyclopedia.com/Pa-St/Sclerotherapy-for-Varicose-Veins.html. Accessed April 15, 2010.
4. Weiss R, Goldman M. Laser treatment of leg veins. Available at: http://emedicine.medscape.com/article/1085867-overview. Accessed April 15, 2010.

Liposuction

Marco A. Pelosi III, MD, FICS[a,b,c,d,e],*,
Marco A. Pelosi II, MD, FICS[b,c,d,e]

KEYWORDS
- Liposuction • Lipoplasty • Suction lipectomy • Aesthetic
- Cosmetic • Body contouring

LIPOSUCTION

The surgical removal of subcutaneous fat using a blunt cannula attached to a suction device is termed *liposuction*. Synonymous terms include *suction lipectomy* and *suction-assisted lipectomy* (SAL). *Lipoplasty*, a broader term, defines any procedure that alters the contours of subcutaneous fat deposits through either removal or addition of fat (liposuction and autologous fat transfer are both examples of lipoplasty). *Lipolysis* reflects the direct ablation of adipocytes using any method.

Liposuction is the most commonly performed cosmetic surgical procedure worldwide. Among North American women, it is second only to breast augmentation in popularity.[1] Currently, indications for liposuction are purely cosmetic, with this procedure having no apparent medical benefit. Frequently treated areas include the torso, extremities, and submandibular regions.

HISTORY

Liposuction evolved from blind sharp excisional procedures. In 1929, Charles Dujarrier, a French surgeon attempted the first contouring procedure of the inner thigh fat deposits, introducing a sharp curette subcutaneously through a small skin incision.[2] Tragically, hemorrhage ensued and the case ended with amputation. Although blinded sharp excisional procedures were revisited several times in subsequent decades with various devices, they were abandoned uniformly because of bleeding-related complications. Giorgio Fischer, an Italian gynecologist, introduced suction as an adjunct to sharp curettage in the mid-1970s.[3]

The authors have nothing to disclose.
[a] Obstetrics & Gynecology, International College of Surgeons-United States Section, Chicago, IL, USA
[b] American Academy of Cosmetic Surgery, Chicago, IL, USA
[c] American Society of Liposuction Surgery, Chicago, IL, USA
[d] International Society of Cosmetogynecology, Bayonne, NJ, USA
[e] Pelosi Medical Center, 350 Kennedy Boulevard, Bayonne, NJ 07002, USA
* Corresponding author. Pelosi Medical Center, 350 Kennedy Boulevard, Bayonne, NJ 07002.
E-mail address: mpelosi3@pelosimedicalcenter.com

Obstet Gynecol Clin N Am 37 (2010) 507–519
doi:10.1016/j.ogc.2010.09.004
0889-8545/10/$ – see front matter © 2010 Elsevier Inc. All rights reserved.

Ives Gerard Illouz of France introduced the first technique of modern liposuction in the late 1970s.[4] Unlike his predecessors, Illouz used blunt suction cannulae and high-powered suction to dislodge and remove subcutaneous fat. The technique used 10-mm cannulae and general endotracheal anesthesia. However, it was associated with significant blood loss, which became the limiting factor in the extent of surgery performed. The technique was later termed *dry liposuction*, reflecting the fact that no fluids were injected into the targeted fat layers before suctioning. Subsequent modifications to the technique included the instillation of a small volume of saline, with or without hyaluronidase, into the fat layer as a lubricant to facilitate cannula motion; this became known as *wet liposuction*. Pierre Fournier, a surgeon trained by Illouz, introduced syringe liposuction and syringe transplantation of the extracted fat. He coined the term *liposculpture* to describe his system.[5] Further refinement of the wet liposuction technique, introduced by Gregory Hetter of Las Vegas in the early 1980s, involved the addition of epinephrine as a vasoconstrictor to the wetting solution.[6]

The mid-1980s marked the modern era of hemostatic liposuction techniques. Central to these methods was the instillation of larger volumes of fluid with epinephrine into the targeted fat layers. Jeffrey Klein, an American dermatologist, introduced a purely local anesthesia technique termed *tumescent liposuction* in 1985.[7] Klein's technique used lidocaine in larger volumes and higher total doses, and smaller caliber cannulae than were used previously, and continues to have the best safety profile of any method of liposuction surgery. Superwet liposuction, also introduced in the mid-1980s, is a technique using general or regional anesthesia in conjunction with lower volumes and concentrations of lidocaine solution than tumescent liposuction. It displays excellent hemostasis and a degree of postoperative analgesia, but carries the risks associated with general or regional anesthesia.

Patient Selection and Assessment

The best candidates for liposuction are physically fit, weight stable, and nonobese, displaying localized adiposity and minimal skin laxity (**Figs. 1** and **2**). They should be classified as ASA1 or ASA2 according to the American Society of Anesthesiologists Physical Status classification system. The tolerance for morbidity is much lower for cosmetic surgery than for therapeutic procedures. Surgeons must keep in mind that

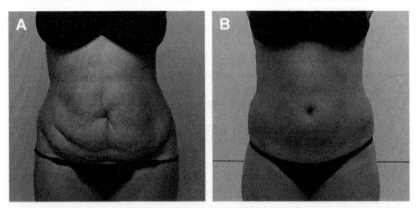

Fig. 1. (A) Patient displaying severe skin laxity, wrinkling, and striae; a poor liposuction candidate. (B) Patient displaying localized abdomen and flanks adiposity with excellent skin tone; an appropriate liposuction candidate.

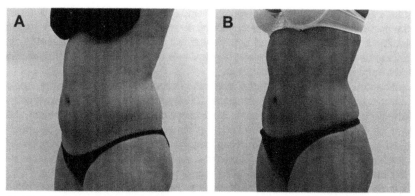

Fig. 2. (A) Patient before and (B) 9 weeks after liposuction of the abdomen and flanks.

the financial burden of any unplanned medical intervention arising from a cosmetic operation typically is not covered by conventional medical insurance. Patients in suboptimal health and those requiring intense perioperative surveillance are not good prospects for this type of surgery.

The localized adiposity to be addressed with surgery should be assessed with the patient standing alongside the surgeon before a full-length mirror, with all relevant areas exposed to allow the patient to explain the cosmetic concerns with precision. Because subcutaneous fat is relatively mobile, the supine position will often yield an inaccurate assessment. Surgeons must point out to patients that cellulite, stretch marks, and significant skin laxity will not be improved with liposuction. Photography is helpful in helping patients view their bodies from multiple perspectives and in defining and explaining the treatment options. Markings are useful in defining the boundaries of proposed treatments and calling attention to preexisting untargeted contour irregularities at both consultation and surgery (**Fig. 3**).

A complete documented medical evaluation should precede any surgery in patients who have not had a recent examination. Any anatomic distortion (eg, hernias) that has the potential to increase the risk for injury should be assessed and managed appropriately before surgery. Blood work analyses include testing for signs of infection,

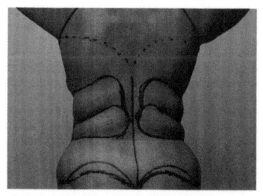

Fig. 3. Markings made in the standing position define the boundaries of proposed treatments and indicate preexisting and untargeted contour irregularities.

anemia, coagulopathy, and liver disease. Pregnancy testing is performed or repeated on the day of surgery irrespective of history. If the physician performing the medical evaluation is not the surgeon and is unfamiliar with liposuction, basic relevant details of the planned anesthetic agents and surgical interventions should be provided along with the request for medical clearance.

Medications, supplements, herbs, and other substances that can impair coagulation should be discontinued before surgery. Substances that interact negatively with anesthetic agents and perioperative medications should also be withheld. If they cannot be discontinued or substituted, the surgical plan will need to be modified, delayed, or withheld. Cigarette smoking is not a contraindication to liposuction, but smokers typically display an atrophic dermis and less skin elasticity, which increase the likelihood of postoperative skin wrinkling.

Expectations and motivations must be explored in depth with cosmetic patients. Unrealistic expectations will never be fulfilled by surgery even if executed to perfection by any medical or aesthetic standard. The cosmetic surgery "addict," the "perfectionist," and the patient expecting cosmetic surgery to remedy interpersonal conflicts are examples of misguided personality types that should be screened out at initial consultation. Similarly, patients seeking weight loss are best served through dietary counseling, the implementation of an appropriate exercise program, and, if necessary, bariatric surgery. Liposuction does not generate long-lasting results or significant weight loss in the presence of poor eating habits and physical inactivity.

ANESTHESIA

Liposuction may be performed with local anesthesia with or without sedation, with epidural anesthesia, or with general anesthesia. Each modality has its advantages, disadvantages, inherent risks, and suitability for the unique demands of each operation and patient. In the United States, most liposuction cases use lidocaine-based instillations into the targeted fat layers as the sole anesthetic (tumescent liposuction) or as an adjunct to general anesthesia (superwet liposuction). In Central and South America, the superwet technique is frequently performed with epidural anesthesia. Regardless of technique, the surgical team should be knowledgeable and prepared, and the facility should be equipped to manage all potential adverse drug effects.

Tumescent local anesthesia, as introduced by Klein and as most commonly prepared, consists of lidocaine hydrochloride, sodium bicarbonate, and epinephrine diluted in normal saline. The target concentration of lidocaine varies depending on the expected sensitivity of the surgical site, but varies little among patients. The target volume of tumescent anesthesia at the surgical site is neither a fixed number nor a fixed ratio of fluid to estimated fat volume; it is determined by the achievement of palpable tumescence (uniform swelling) of the field, which is determined, in turn, by the elasticity, density, and size of the targeted fat deposit. The maximum safe dose of tumescent local anesthesia is based on the amount of lidocaine administered. Most surgeons consider a lidocaine dose of 50 mg/kg to be the toxicity threshold for tumescent anesthesia for liposuction. Lidocaine administered in this fashion displays a peak serum level 12 hours postinfiltration, and complete elimination by 36 hours postinfiltration; it is metabolized through the liver primarily through the cytochrome p450 system.[8]

Superwet liposuction uses an instillation of the same ingredients as tumescent local anesthesia, albeit at a much lower concentration of lidocaine and a much lower volume, because the surgical anesthesia is conducted using general or epidural modalities. The purpose of superwet infiltration of the targeted fat layers is primarily the hemostasis generated by the epinephrine in the solution, and secondarily the post-operative analgesia produced by the lidocaine. In some instances, no lidocaine is used in the solution.

Both tumescent and superwet liposuction operations begin with the instillation of their respective solutions into the layers of the targeted fat deposit through needle infiltration (**Fig. 4**). The needle may be either a disposable sharp spinal-type needle or a reusable blunt-tipped infusion needle with apertures along the shaft. The infiltration needle may be connected to either a syringe or a pressurized infusion pump system through tubing. The fluid is delivered with a steady fanning motion in horizontal planes, commencing in the deep fat layers and progressing superficially. Because the needle is in constant motion, there is no need to watch for a flashback of blood into the tubing or syringe.

ANATOMY

Subdermal fat throughout the trunk and extremities exists in compartments within a connective tissue matrix termed the superficial fascial system (SFS) that extends from the subdermis to the muscle fascia.[9] The SFS consists of horizontal sheets of membranous connective tissue connected by vertical and oblique septa. Scarpa's fascia of the lower abdomen is an example of a well-defined horizontal sheet of the SFS. In other areas these sheets may be multiple and less distinct. As adiposity increases, the layers of fat within the SFS increase in thickness.[10]

Within each layer, adipose tissue is organized into large visible subunits of varying size, termed *fat pearls*. Fat pearls are composed of smaller ovoid subunits with a pasty consistency known as *fat lobules* and typically are not visible individually without magnification. Fat lobules consist of clusters of adipocytes and are supplied with capillaries and sometimes nerves.[11] Microscopic sections of fat tissue show fibroblast-like preadipocytes, mature adipocytes, and adult stem cells; the latter have the capacity to form muscle and bone.[12]

Techniques

Basic techniques of modern liposuction use steel blunt suction cannulas of diameters ranging from 1 to 10 mm (**Fig. 5**). Cannulas 2 mm or narrower are termed *microcannulae*. Cannulas larger than 5 mm are not commonly used when using purely local anesthesia. Narrower cannulas offer more control, whereas wider cannulas offer faster

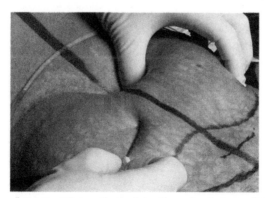

Fig. 4. Infiltration of tumescent anesthesia into the subcutaneous fat performed using a spinal needle.

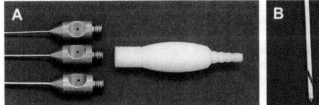
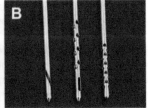

Fig. 5. (*A*) Vented liposuction cannulae of various diameters and a detachable Teflon handle. (*B*) Examples of cannula tip and hole patterns.

extraction. Other design variables include tip configuration, aperture configuration, shaft length, and handle design. Handles may be either fused or detachable and may possess a vacuum vent.

Cannulae are designed to be connected to either suction tubing or syringes. Suction tubing is connected to an aspiration pump, which typically is set to operate at a maximum vacuum pressure of −100 kPa (−750 mm Hg). The pressure is greater than that created by conventional operating room general suction devices, and requires semirigid tubing to resist collapse. When syringes are used, various piston locking mechanisms may be used to minimize hand fatigue.

Small skin incisions serve as entry ports for liposuction cannulae. These incisions are most commonly made with either skin punches or a scalpel and whenever possible are hidden within bikini lines, skin folds, scars, or tattoos (**Fig. 6**). Skin punch incisions are preferred when surgeons want the sites to remain open for postoperative drainage.

The process of liposuction necessitates a back and forth motion of the cannula as suction simultaneously holds fat tissue in the lateral apertures of the cannula shaft. This action results in the avulsion of small parcels of fat from its connective tissue attachments, creating tunnels through this matrix along the paths taken by the instrument. Tunneling creates narrow channels devoid of fat that collapse under the weight of the overlying tissue and is the mechanism through which contouring is achieved. The process typically does not damage blood vessels and nerves because they offer greater resistance to avulsion and because the cannula apertures do not have sharpened edges. The combination of fat and fluid removed as a result of this process is

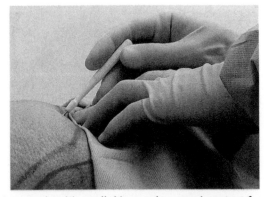

Fig. 6. Access incisions made with small skin punches remain patent for several days, facilitating passive drainage of tissue fluids and minimizing edema.

termed the *lipoaspirate*, and over time it can be observed in the collection canister to separate into a yellow supernatant fat layer and a blood-tinged infranatant fluid layer (**Fig. 7**). When the back and forth cannula action is generated exclusively by the motion of the surgeon's hand, the process is called *manual liposuction*. When the cannula action is generated by a motorized handle, the process is known as *power-assisted liposuction* (PAL).

Control over the direction of the liposuction cannula is the cornerstone of both safety and an adequate cosmetic result. The nondominant hand plays a central role in this process through continuously confirming depth and direction, and detecting and protecting vital local anatomy. Under most circumstances, the motion of the cannula is parallel to the underlying muscle fascia and the process proceeds in horizontal planes starting in the deeper fat layers (**Fig. 8**).

The end point of the liposuction process is variable and determined by a combination of the patient's wishes, the nature of the skin and fat layers, underlying musculoskeletal architecture, and the need to develop symmetry. For example, when treating the inner or outer thigh fat deposits, a relatively large amount of fat intentionally is left behind to preserve the characteristic female contours, whereas when treating the abdomen, very little fat is preserved to enhance the definition of muscle lines. Total extirpation of the subcutaneous fat is never the goal of the procedure, and if pursued is likely to produce irreversible and unsightly injury to the overlying skin. It is prudent to leave the first 5 mm of superficial subdermal fat intact as a way to protect the delicate subdermal vascular plexus and minimize the risk of dermal trauma, which most frequently manifests as skin wrinkling. At surgery, the thickness of the subcutaneous fat layers is determined by pinching them between the fingertips as the fat deposits are gradually debulked.

The upper limit of fat volume that may safely be removed in a single liposuction session has not yet been defined by science, but in some instances has been constrained by law. For example, in California, extracting more than 5000 mL total aspirate volume per procedure outside of an acute care hospital is deemed unprofessional (SB 450 Speier Bill, adopted August 31, 1999), and in Florida, exceeding 4000 mL total fat aspirate volume in tumescent liposuction procedures is prohibited in an office surgical facility (64B89–9.009, Standard of Care for Office

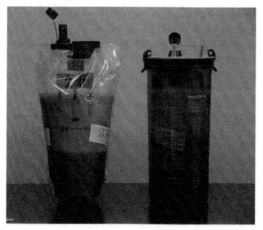

Fig. 7. The lipoaspirate separates into a supernatant layer of fat and an infranatant layer of blood-tinged fluid.

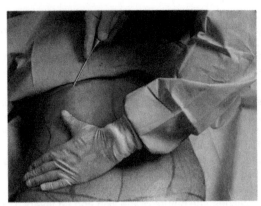

Fig. 8. Control of the liposuction cannula is achieved with the nondominant hand, which defines depth, direction and the boundaries of local anatomy. Cannula motion is parallel to the underlying muscle fascia.

Surgery, adopted February 17, 2000). In practical terms, purely tumescent liposuction is limited inherently by lidocaine dosing constraints. Nonetheless, it would be difficult to assert that the removal of a fixed volume of fat produces the same degree of surgical trauma in people of vastly different size and whether removed from a single area or multiple sites.

Perioperative Care

Because liposuction involves extensive manipulation of skin structures, broad-spectrum antibiotic prophylaxis targeting common skin pathogens is used either orally or parenterally immediately before surgery. The skin is cleansed with the same agents used for conventional therapeutic surgery. When surgery is performed totally using local anesthesia, noninvasive monitoring of blood pressure, electrocardiogram, and pulse oximetry parameters is routine.

After surgery, absorbent dressings are placed over all incision sites; drainage of serosanguineous fluid from unsutured incision sites typically ceases in 2 to 3 days. Compression garments are applied over the wound dressings and over the complete span of each surgical site. High-compression (ie, "phase one") garments are worn continuously until drainage from the incision sites ceases. Lower-compression (ie, "phase two") garments are worn continuously thereafter for 4 to 6 weeks. Rarely is postoperative discomfort severe. Most patients describe varying degrees of a burning soreness over the muscle layer at the treatment sites that responds well to nonsteroidal anti-inflammatory medications. Massage of the treatment sites frequently expedites resolution of varying degrees of soft tissue swelling common after this type of surgery. No established standards exist for postliposuction massage, but most regimens begin a minimum of 2 weeks after surgery, when the patient's discomfort level from this type of therapy is low. Complete healing and tissue remodeling require approximately 6 months. Within this timeframe, induration of the treatment sites develops and resolves.

Complications

Complications may relate to either anesthesia or surgery. Anesthetic complications of general and regional anesthesia are no different for liposuction than for other types of surgery. However, the addition of large volumes of superwet or tumescent fluids into the fat layers creates the potential added risk of fluid overload if the patient is receiving significant amounts of intravenous fluid simultaneously. When liposuction is performed totally using local tumescent anesthesia, intravenous access is established only for the purpose of administering medications; fluids are administered orally, intermittently, and in small volumes.

Lidocaine overdose is rare with tumescent liposuction when toxicity thresholds are assessed and respected, but patients taking medications that interfere with lidocaine metabolism are at increased risk. Allergic reactions to the components of tumescent and superwet solutions have been described in their undiluted states and are most commonly attributed to preservatives such as sodium metabisulfite. Allergies to lidocaine hydrochloride, an amide anesthetic, are rare.[13]

Visceral and vascular perforation injuries from either infusion needles or liposuction cannulae are rare. They have been reported in association with surgery in the presence of an abdominal scar or hernia and with large-volume cases under general anesthesia.[14,15]

Surgically related thromboembolism is a function of venous stasis, endothelial injury, and hypercoagulability. These conditions are more characteristic of prolonged procedures performed under general anesthesia or deep sedation than tumescent local anesthesia, but nonsurgical factors such as oral contraceptive use, inherited coagulation disorders, a history of smoking, or a long trip spent sitting in a car or an airplane perioperatively should alert the surgeon to the need for mechanical or pharmacologic prophylaxis irrespective of the type of anesthesia used.

Fat embolism, which occurs asymptomatically in most cases of orthopedic trauma, is distinct from fat embolism syndrome (FES) which is relatively rare and rarer still in relation to liposuction.[14,15] FES is a delayed biochemical inflammatory condition which, when severe, is marked by respiratory distress, cerebral dysfunction, and a petechial rash 24 to 48 hours after surgery. Emboli of fat may also provoke mechanical blockage of the pulmonary capillaries, resulting in tachycardia, tachypnea, elevated temperature, hypoxemia, hypocapnia, thrombocytopenia, and mild neurologic symptoms.[16]

Hemorrhage from direct vascular injury within the surgical field is not typically seen with either tumescent or superwet liposuction because of the vasoconstriction that both of these modalities produce. Low-level intraoperative bleeding is sometimes provoked by venturing beyond the zone of vasoconstriction, from either inadvertently venturing into fat outside the treatment zone or grazing the underlying superficial layers of muscle and fascia with the cannula. The latter respond well to compression and targeted infiltrations of dilute epinephrine. Case reports of significant bleeding necessitating blood transfusion during liposuction indicate deep tissue lacerations and perforations under general anesthesia or deep sedation.

Bruising, typically mild, is common after liposuction, but less so when small-caliber cannulae, pure tumescent techniques, and drainage are used (**Fig. 9**). Not infrequently, bruising will appear in areas dependent to the surgical field. More extensive bruising accompanies the use of systemic anesthesia, larger instrumentation, and the treatment of highly vascular regions, such as the submandibular fat pad and the breast. Hypertensive patients are at higher risk for bruising.

Hematomas and seromas are uncommon in liposuction, but when seen are usually related to the treatment of richly vascularized areas, such as the breast or the submental fat pad, and may be associated with extensive bruising. Sonography is a useful assessment tool for these conditions. Primary treatment in both instances is drainage and compression. Hematomas left undrained subcutaneously provoke wrinkling of the overlying skin.

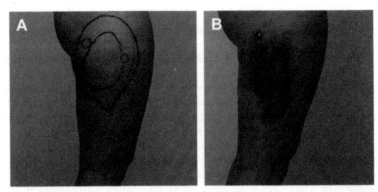

Fig. 9. (A) The right outer thigh of a 26-year-old patient is shown before and (B) 11 days after liposuction showing moderate bruising. She noted no particular discomfort.

Infection is rare with this type of surgery, probably because of the selection of exclusively healthy patients, the common use of dedicated clean operating rooms, antibiotic prophylaxis, and the routine use of postoperative drainage. The common method of postliposuction drainage is through the egress of fluid from unsutured cannula sites rather than by the placement of indwelling drains. Necrotizing fasciitis, the most dangerous type of tissue infection, has been reported with liposuction, is most commonly caused by streptococcus pyogenes, and is extremely rare.[17]

Partial- or full-thickness skin necrosis **Fig. 10** can occur when the vascular supply to the skin is injured through various means. Damage may be provoked by excessively superficial liposuction, pressure from improperly worn compression garments, ice packs, infection, and dermal atrophy, which is common with obesity, advancing age, and chronic cigarette smoking. Prompt and regular debridement with either sharp instrumentation or hydrogen peroxide and appropriate antibiotic coverage until healthy granulation tissue develops are the mainstays of management. Lesser degrees of vascular injury to the dermis manifest as areas of erythematous skin discoloration.

Contour irregularities subsequent to liposuction may range from mild to severe. Proper positioning and surgical technique minimize these defects, but when they occur they can be managed with either autologous fat transfer (sometimes referred to as *lipofilling*) or liposhifting. Autologous fat transfer involves the harvest of fat through liposuction from areas usually remote from the intended recipient site, separation of the fat from the anesthetic fluids, and fine incremental injection of the purified fat in layers into the targeted region using small syringes and blunt-tipped fat transfer cannulae. Numerous techniques are available for separating and preparing the harvested fat, but are beyond the scope of this article. With liposhifting, the fat peripheral

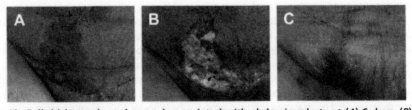

Fig. 10. Full-thickness dermal necrosis associated with abdominoplasty at (A) 6 days, (B) 13 days, and (C) 12 weeks.

to an iatrogenic concavity is loosened through mechanical disruption using specialized cannulae and then massaged vigorously into the target area.[18]

Technology

Liposuction is most commonly performed manually and generally produces excellent results in properly selected patients. Nonetheless, the process is tedious and requires prolonged repetitive motion by surgeon. Consequently, one of the major stimuli for technological innovation has been to facilitate the liposuction process.

Liposuction has been found to require less time and effort when the integrity of the targeted fat layers has been partially disrupted, especially in the presence of fibrous tissue, scar tissue, or a previously liposuctioned field. Three methods are approved by the U.S. Food and Drug Association to achieve this goal: mechanical disruption, internal ultrasound, and external laser therapy. All require preliminary tumescent or superwet infiltration of the fat layers.

Slow mechanical disruption of the fat layers using smooth cannulae without suction was originally described as a way to soften the transition between the treatment site and the surrounding tissues during wet liposuction, and was termed *mesh undermining* in the early 1980s.[19] The process was subsequently adopted as a pretreatment of the targeted fat during wet liposuction and found to facilitate both cannula motion and the achievement of smooth contours, and dubbed *pretunneling*.[20] Pretunneling reemerged as "fat disruption" in 2003, a pretreatment to tumescent liposuction with the goal of speeding the surgical process.[21] Unlike its predecessor, fat disruption uses cannulae with flared apertures originally designed for liposhifting, which are more effective at softening the tissues of the SFS than are smooth cannulae.

Internal ultrasonic emulsification of the targeted fat layers was introduced in 1987.[22] Termed *ultrasound-assisted liposuction* (UAL), this technology uses metallic probes to deliver mechanical vibrations at frequencies ranging from 20 to 60 kHz, which interact with the targeted tissues through direct thermal effects, cavitation, and direct mechanical effects. The emulsified fat is then removed through conventional liposuction. Burn injuries continue to plague this modality because ultrasonic energy can easily turn into heat energy (ie, the widely used harmonic scalpel uses the same basic principles exclusively for their thermal effects). An external version of this technology using skin paddles and a gel interface was introduced in the 1990s, but no device is currently on the market.[23] Other adaptions of external ultrasound technology that bypass the need to use liposuction are marketed outside the United States, but remain a topic of continued investigation.[24]

A technique of external laser-assisted liposuction was introduced in 2000.[25] The procedure, termed *low-level laser-assisted lipoplasty*, used a 635-nm, 10 mW diode laser applied in conjunction with tumescent anesthesia before conventional liposuction. The authors showed microscopically that the laser action caused transient pores to open in the adipocytes cell membrane, allowing its contents to move into the interstitial space. They commented that the latter effect resulted in easier fat extraction and less surgical trauma and bruising. An attempt to duplicate these microscopic findings by another group using superwet rather than tumescent solution was unsuccessful.[26]

Powered liposuction cannulae offer a more direct alternative for reducing surgical fatigue but do not reduce operating time to any perceivable degree. Power-assisted liposuction (PAL) devices became available in 2000.[27] Various designs include electric motors, pneumatic motors, axial motion, rotational motion, and oscillation. Patients typically perceive less discomfort with PAL cannulae because of their inherent vibration when activated. PAL is sometimes referred to as *vibroliposuction*.

Aside from facilitating the liposuction process, various technologies have focused on augmenting the benefits of the procedure. Internal laser devices for assisting conventional liposuction surgery were first described in 1992,[28] with the implication that laser-mediated coagulation of blood vessels, collagen, and adipocytes would result in less blood loss, bruising, and tissue reorganization. First-generation devices were low-energy 1065-nm neodymium:yttrium-aluminum-garnet lasers and were heavily marketed in South America and subsequently in North America, but clinical studies, including a prospective randomized trial comparing it to standard liposuction, failed to find any major cosmetic or convalescent differences.[29] Lasers continue to flood the liposuction market, touting "unique" combinations of wavelengths and wattages, each promising the ultimate cosmetic results with little more than the anecdotal blessing of a handful of industry-friendly surgeons. Water-assisted liposuction was introduced in Europe in 2005, with the promise of less tissue trauma, using a powered cannula that delivers a pulsatile flow of fluid and aspirates simultaneously,[30–32] but data are insufficient to substantiate whether the procedure offers any advantages over existing methods in terms of complications or cosmesis.

SUMMARY

Liposuction provides effective contouring of the torso, extremities, and submental areas in properly selected patients. Effective techniques have been established for performing liposuction under local anesthesia and general anesthesia. Both methods share many similarities regarding the surgical craft of fat removal, but have distinct elements of anesthetic precaution that must be respected to optimize safety. No technology seems to give superior results over conventional methods.

REFERENCES

1. Cosmetic Surgery National Data Bank. 2008 Statistics. New York (NY): American Society for Aesthetic Plastic Surgery; 2009. p. 3.
2. Comiskey C. Cosmetic surgery in Paris in 1926: the case of the amputated leg. J Wom Hist 2004;16(3):30–54.
3. Fischer A, Fischer GM. Revised technique for cellulitis fat reduction in riding breeches deformity. Bull Int Acad Cosmetic Surg 1977;2:40.
4. Illouz YG. Une nouvelle technique pour les lipodystrophies localisées. La Revue de Chirurgie Esthétique de Langue Française 1980;6(19):10–2.
5. Fournier P. Liposculpture: ma technique. Paris: Librairie Arnette; 1990.
6. Hetter GP. The effect of low-dose epinephrine on the hematocrit drop following lipolysis. Aesthetic Plast Surg 1984;8(1):19–21.
7. Klein JA. Tumescent technique for liposuction surgery. Am J Cosm Surg 1987;4: 263–7.
8. Klein JA. Tumescent technique for regional anesthesia permits lidocaine doses of 35 mg/kg for liposuction. J Dermatol Surg Oncol 1990;16:248–63.
9. Lockwood TE. Superficial fascial system (SFS) of the trunk and extremities: a new concept. Plast Reconstr Surg 1991;87(6):1009–18.
10. Avelar J. Regional distribution and behavior of the subcutaneous tissue concerning selection and indication for liposuction. Aesthetic Plast Surg 1989;13(3): 155–65.
11. Klein JA. Subcutaneous fat: anatomy and histology. Tumescent technique: tumescent anesthesia and microcannular liposuction. Philadelphia: Mosby; 2000. p. 213–21.

12. Kaminski M, Lopez deVaughn RM. The anatomy and physiology metabolism/ nutrition of subcutaneous fat. In: Shiffman MA, DiGiuseppe A, editors. Liposuction: principles and practice. Berlin: Springer; 2006. p. 17–25.

13. Gonzalez-Delgado P, Antón R, Soriano V, et al. Cross-reactivity among amide-type local anesthetics in a case of allergy to mepivacaine. J Investig Allergol Clin Immunol 2006;16:311–3.

14. Talmor M, Hoffman IA, Lieberman M. Intestinal perforation after suction lipoplasty: a case report and review of the literature. Aesthetic Plast Surg 1997;38:169–72.

15. Shiffman MA. Prevention and treatment of liposuction complications. In: Shiffman MA, DiGiuseppe A, editors. Liposuction: principles and practice. Berlin: Springer; 2006. p. 333–41.

16. Levy D. The fat embolism syndrome: a review. Clin Orthop 1990;261:281–6.

17. Wang HD, Zheng JH, Deng CL, et al. Fat embolism syndromes following liposuction. Aesthetic Plast Surg 2008;32:731–6.

18. Haeck PC, Swanson JA, Gutowski KA, et al. Evidence-based patient safety advisory: liposuction. Plast Reconstr Surg 2009;124:28S–44S.

19. Heitman C, Czermak C, German G. Rapidly fatal necrotizing fasciitis after aesthetic liposuction. Aesthetic Plast Surg 2000;24:344–7.

20. Saylan Z. Liposhifting instead of lipofilling: treatment of postlipoplasty irregularities. Aesthet Surg J 2001;21:137–41.

21. Hetter GP. Surgical technique. In: Hetter GP, editor. Lipoplasty: the theory and practice of blunt suction lipectomy. Boston: Little, Brown and Co; 1984. p.137–54.

22. Mladick RA, Morris RL. Alternative patient positioning and pretunneling. In: Hetter GP, editor. Lipoplasty: the theory and practice of blunt suction lipectomy. Boston: Little, Brown and Co; 1984. p.137–54.

23. Mangubat EA. Fat disruption using the Blugerman liposhifting instrument. Philadelphia: American Academy of Cosmetic Surgery Fall Symposium on Body Augmentation and Contouring; October 2003.

24. Scuderi N, de Vita R, d'Andrea F, et al. Nuove prospettive nella liposuzione: la lipoemulsificazione. Giorn Chir Plast Ricostr Estet 1987;2:1.

25. Rosenberg GJ, Cabrera RC. External ultrasonic lipoplasty: an effective method of fat removal and skin shrinkage. Plast Reconstr Surg 2000;105:785–91.

26. Brown SA, Greenbaum L, Shtukmaster S, et al. Characterization of nonthermal focused ultrasound for noninvasive selective fat cell destruction (lysis). Plast Reconstr Surg 2009;124:92–101.

27. Neira R, Arroyave J, Ramirez H, et al. Fat liquefaction: effect of low-level laser energy on adipose tissue. Plast Reconstr Surg 2000;110:912–22.

28. Brown SA, Rohrich RJ, Kenkel J, et al. Effect of low-level laser therapy on abdominal adipocytes before lipoplasty procedures. Plast Reconstr Surg 2004;113:1796–804.

29. Coleman WP III. Powered liposuction. Dermatol Surg 2000;26:315–8.

30. Apfelberg D. Laser-assisted liposuction may benefit surgeons and subjects. Clin Laser Mon 1992;10:259.

31. Prado A, Andrades P, Danilla S, et al. A prospective, randomized, double-blind, controlled clinical trial comparing laser-assisted lipoplasty with suction-assisted lipoplasty. Plast Reconstr Surg 2006;118:1032–45.

32. Araco A, Gravante G, Araco F, et al. Comparison of power water-assisted and traditional liposuction: a prospective randomized trial of postoperative pain. Aesthetic Plast Surg 2007;31:259–65.

The Use of Autologous Fat for Facial Rejuvenation

Benjamin C. Marcus, MD

KEYWORDS

- Autologous fat • Grafting • Facial rejuvenation
- Fat injectionhead

There is no doubt what a youthful face looks like. A glance at a child shows skin that is smooth and flawless, with no telltale sign of gravity's pull (**Fig. 1**). As one ages, skin becomes lax and muscles and deeper tissue slip from their positions (**Fig. 2**). Why is it then that most facial aesthetic procedures focus on just tightening the facial skin and lifting the sagging structures? Clearly, a youthful face is an additional benefit to those who seek to reverse the signs of aging. Aging may be likened to turning of a grape into a raisin. Facelifts alone just smooth out the raisin. To really transform a raisin back into a grape, volume needs to be added to the face.

Adding volume to the aging face is a notion that has lately come into vogue but is, however, not a new idea. The use of fat for volumetric enhancement of the face dates back to the 1890s.[1] Earlier, harvests were done en bloc and had success in some limited applications. The use of bulky segments of abdominal fat is ill suited, at least for selective volume enhancement of the face.

With the advent of liposuction techniques, there is renewed interest in the use of aspirated fat. The fat obtained by standard liposuction proved to be difficult to graft successfully because of the size of the harvested adipocytes and the technique with which fat was injected. Over the last 10 years, there have been great advances in the techniques of harvest and grafting. There has also been advancement in the instrumentation available to allow for a more consistent technique.

Commercial fillers have a valuable place in the cosmetic surgeon's armamentarium.[2] Not all patients look for long-term results from a fat transfer, and others may want a less-invasive procedure without the need for a fat aspiration. Commercial fillers offer immediate volume correction with a more modest financial commitment. Nevertheless, the standardization of fat grafting techniques, with the ability to correct all aspects of the aging face with safe, natural, and lasting results, marks an exciting article in facial aesthetics.

Division of Otolaryngology, Department of Surgery, University of Wisconsin–Madison, 600 Highland Avenue, BX 7375 Clinical Science Center-H4, Madison, WI 53792-3284, USA
E-mail address: marcus@surgery.wisc.edu

Obstet Gynecol Clin N Am 37 (2010) 521–531
doi:10.1016/j.ogc.2010.10.003
0889-8545/10/$ – see front matter © 2010 Elsevier Inc. All rights reserved.

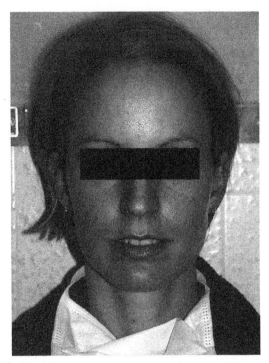

Fig. 1. A youthful face.

THE PHYSIOLOGY OF THE AGING FACE

There is no doubt that the aging face is changed by gravity. As one ages, some of the key architectural elements of skin, such as collagen and elastin, are lost. Photoaging also occurs, and the cumulative exposure of the facial skin to the sun further robs it of the earlier structural stability. An often overlooked aspect of facial aging is the thinning of the subcutaneous layer of facial fat. This layer is an essential scaffold that helps hold the facial skin envelope in its original youthful position. As this layer thins, there is an element of pseudoptosis that accentuates the genuine ptosis that is engendered from the concomitant loss of collagen and elastin.[3]

The case for facial fat as a key element of the youthful face can be furthered by observing certain disease states that promote an early or accelerated loss of facial fat. In cases such as scleroderma, localized loss of fat produces a more aged appearance.[4] Lipoatrophy caused by antiretroviral therapy for human immunodeficiency virus infection is even more prevalent in the modern age. Long-term therapy with these lifesaving drugs produces a characteristic loss of facial fat that is quite pronounced and gives these patients a prematurely aged and sickly appearance.[5]

HISTORY OF FAT AS A FILLER

The history of fat grafting dates back to the nineteenth century. In the 1890s,[6] fat grafts were harvested as a whole and directly transferred for augmentation. The process of injecting fat began in the 1920s.[7] Despite existing in the armamentarium of surgeons for more than 100 years, the technique of fat grafting has gained popularity only during the last 20 years. This gain in popularity may be, in part, because of the concomitant

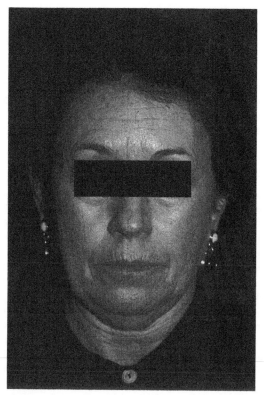

Fig. 2. The face as it ages.

increase in the performance of liposuction. A large supply of aspirated fat makes the surgeon use this material. Another reason for the long period between inception and acceptance is the uncertainty of the long-term survival of the grafted material.

Early work in the 1920s sought to use grafted fat in the periocular region for the repair of tuberculosis-related scarring. This work showed some early promise because the fat was a good match for the contour defect. However, over time, the volume of the fat grafts diminished.[8] Further work showed that the volume loss was related to central necrosis of the transplanted fat, which was thought to be related to the inadequate blood supply that the host tissue was able to produce. The peripheral fat cells seemed to be viable.[9] This discovery led to the postulate that fat should be transplanted in small volumes to allow for proper revascularization.

Nearly a quarter of a century later, additional research provided a set of contradictory findings. Peer[10] evaluated fat grafts in both human and animal settings. The experiments showed that at least half of the transplanted fat would be lost in the first year. Furthermore, this loss could be continuous, leading to eventual dissolution of the fat graft. In contradiction to earlier reports, this research also showed that the center rather than the periphery of the graft was the portion that was most likely to survive. This midcentury work led to the decline in interest of the surgical community in autologous fat grafting.

The last 15 to 20 years have witnessed a gradual increase in the interest in facial fat grafting, which may be related to the increased understanding of the role that fillers play in facial rejuvenation. For example, from the late 1990s till today, there has been a significant increase in the use of commercial fillers, such as Juvederm and Radiesse.[11] It is natural that cosmetic practitioners look for truly autologous fillers that can be used to further these same goals. Another reason for the renewed interest in fat grafting is the advancements in the harvest and preparation techniques for fat transfer. Coleman advanced a technique he termed "structural" fat grafting, which focused on an atraumatic harvest method, centrifugation for purification, and specific injection techniques. This technique is detailed later in the article. Coleman[12] was able to show an improved rate of fat graft survival and a high rate of patient satisfaction. His published results also heralded a renewed interest in this method (**Fig. 3**).

HARVEST AND STORAGE TECHNIQUES
Site of Harvest

There are multiple sources for fat grafting material. Abundant fat is found in the abdomen, thighs, or buttocks. Each of these locations is easily accessed in the office or operating room setting. Aspirated fat is also incidentally harvested during facial rejuvenation surgery, such as facelifts and submental liposuction. It is not yet clear if there is any difference in the physiology of the fat depending on its origin because fat from the head and neck would better suit the facial region than fat from the abdomen. Fat grafted to the breasts might also function better if its origin was the trunk. However, only very few studies addressed this topic. A review of practice patterns demonstrated that the most common site of fat harvest was the abdomen because it is an easily accessed area and often has ample material for harvest.[13]

The study by Rohrich and colleagues[14] is one of the few studies that addressed the site of origin and fat cell viability. The investigators analyzed the fat harvested from a variety of body sites and determined cell viability with standard spectrophotometric analysis. The analysis showed no statistical difference between the sites of harvest.

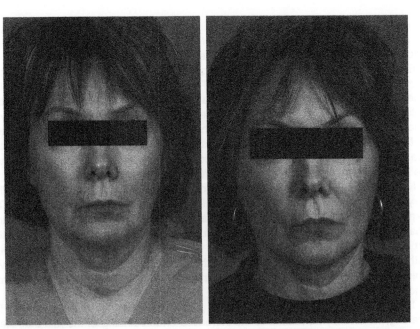

Fig. 3. A face before (*left*) and after (*right*) autologous fat grafting.

A limitation of the study was the ex vivo nature of the analysis. Subtle differences in survival might be elucidated if the quantification occurred in the engrafted site. Further studies in this area would be valuable if an advantage for a particular harvest site could be demonstrated for facial procedures.

Harvest Techniques

As is the case with many aspects of the autologous fat grafting technique, there is significant disparity in the evidence for the ideal harvest technique. There are essentially 3 major types of harvest technique: (1) aspiration of fat microparticles, (2) harvest of fat cores, and (3) direct microexcision. There is evidence to support each of these techniques. Aspiration of fat microparticles is the most common technique. This technique centers on the use of already available liposuction equipment, which is appealing to most practitioners. It is thought that the harvest of small fat bundles allows for easy reinjection and promotes a more successful ingrowth of vascularization at the donor site. Using a small-gauge cannula alone is not sufficient to promote viability of the harvested fat. Small-gauge cannulas that are used with high-pressure suction systems can result in up to 90% cell death compared with those used with low-power suction aspirators.[15] The lower-pressure technique is performed using the same small-gauge cannula, but the suction provided is from a manually controlled syringe. An underreported advantage of this technique is that it does not rely on expensive liposuction hardware and can easily be performed in the office setting with a minimal capital outlay.

The harvest of fat cores has also been promoted. This method suggests that fat cells are damaged by the aspiration technique and have a better rate of survival when they are harvested in a series of intact cores. The comparison was performed in an animal model, which showed that the aspirated fat had a poorer overall survival rate.[16] Although the measurements performed were volumetric, there was no specific physiologic mechanism elucidated for these findings. One might postulate that the intact cores of fat had a better network of microcirculation. Alternatively, the fat cells themselves may suffer less damage during the harvest process. The cores of fat are suitable for injection in many areas of the face but have limited use in the areas of the face that require nuanced volume replacement (such as the periocular region).

The final major technique of fat harvest is direct excision. In facial rejuvenation, this technique centers on the use of incidentally harvested fat during other rejuvenation techniques, such as rhytidectomy. Fat from the submentum or excess skin can be reduced and directly implanted. It is less common to harvest the fat from an alternative site, such as the abdomen, because of the need for an additional incision site. Harvested fat behaves in a manner different from that of the traditional dermal fat grafts that have been harvested from the abdomen (and elsewhere) because they lack the supporting vascular architecture in the accompanying dermis. There are multiple proponents of small fat pearls for surgical implantation. Many of the strongest arguments for this technique are seen in the oculoplastic literature.[17] In these cases, small intact pearls of fat are used for adding volume to the upper and lower lid structures. These pearls of fat are used for primary augmentation and secondary correction of previous surgery. The major difference in the augmentation of the lid structures is the ease of making an incision for the direct implantation of the grafts. This type of direct surgical placement would be impractical in other areas of the face.

Preservation Techniques

One of the main obstacles in using fat as a filling agent is the concern of reabsorption. Regardless of the harvest technique and purification protocols, some of the injected fat does not survive. Analysis has shown up to a 50% loss of engrafted fat with long-term follow-up.[18] Because of the known tissue loss, there is significant interest in cryo-preservation of the harvested fat, which allows for reinjection at later sessions without the need for an additional harvest session.

Early attempts at the long-term storage of fat grafts centered on a simple freezing method without any additional processing. This method resulted in poor adipose cell survival.[19] Later attempts included the use of immediate freezing with liquid nitrogen but were not successful in improving the survival rate of fat. Simple freezing led to up to a 97% loss of viable adipocytes.[20]

A recent study[21] analyzed freezing harvested fat with several novel techniques. After fat was harvested in a standard manner, the investigators used a combination of permeable and nonpermeable cryoprotection agents. The goal of this technique was to avoid the formation of intracellular ice crystals, which lead to cell death. The agents used were permeable and nonpermeable, which provided both intra- and extracellular protection. The freezing protocol was standardized for induction. There were 2 methods of assessing cell viability. The first was a standard histologic analysis, and the second, a biochemical assay. Using the protocol as described, the investigators demonstrated that adipocyte viability was essentially unchanged. The addition of a cryopreservation solution and careful freezing protocol allowed the physician to perform a single fat harvest and have ample material for later injections.

PURIFICATION TECHNIQUES

A comprehensive analysis performed at the author's institution evaluated multiple methods of fat purification. Piasecki and colleagues[22] examined the most common methods and submitted them to a rigorous model for survival analysis. The viability of adipose cells was analyzed with histologic and biochemical markers for survival. Quantitative comparisons were made between blunt and sharp harvests as well as centrifuged and decanted samples. Modest changes were seen in each of these groups, with the blunt harvested and centrifuged samples fairing the best. A more dramatic result was seen when the group added a collagenase treatment to the protocol. With this element in place, they were able to demonstrate ex vivo survival in the mid-90%. Although this study is limited to the ex vivo survival of the fat grafts, it provides a good starting point for best harvest practices that should be further applied in an in vivo model (**Fig. 4**).

An exciting area of investigation is the use of adjuvant therapies to augment the survival of the harvested fat. Because fat survival is paramount to the success of

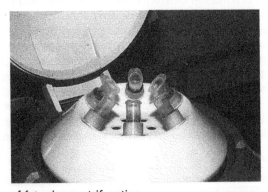

Fig. 4. Preparation of fat using centrifugation.

the procedure, any additional step that can improve fat cell survival would be highly valued. Some investigators, such as Coleman, argue against the addition of growth factors, stating that the native fat is all that is needed for a successful procedure.[21] With the available data, however, there are some promising techniques.

A recently published report showed a significant improvement in the overall graft survival when the fat cells were coincubated with a cocktail of exogenous factors. This study analyzed the addition of nonsteroidal hormones, thyroxin, and other growth factors. The study was a human clinical trial, and a volumetric computed tomographic scan was used to assess survival. Rates of graft take were as high as 90% in some subjects. This level of success is much greater than that in previously published reports. One drawback about this study is that multiple exogenous factors were added in combination, which makes it hard to determine what factors are helpful and what are superfluous. Another confounding factor with this study is the inability to determine what concentration of the factors persists after injection. A clever mechanism of factor delivery was performed in a different study. Drug-eluting microspheres that were included in the injection were used for their animal models.[23] The spheres discharged insulinlike growth factor 1 and basic fibroblast growth factor in many different combinations. When compared with fat injected with the microsphere without these factors, there was significant improvement in cell viability. Although this area of research is exciting, it makes a simple procedure potentially much more complicated and expensive. Therefore, it is not yet clear if the overall improvement in survival in the trials that include exogenous factors validates the use of these factors.

The major barrier for survival of transplanted fat is the lack of adequate oxygenation. In 2000, Shoshani and colleagues[24] looked at the role of hyperbaric oxygen as an adjuvant to fat grafting. They inferred that increasing the partial tension of oxygen in the blood might aid in the survival of the grafts. However, data from this study demonstrated little overall benefit for the technique. Even at levels approaching 2 atm of oxygen for sustained periods there was little overall change in viability. The practicality of this technique has to be questioned even if it were highly successful. Maintaining patients in a hyperbaric oxygen protocol would be prohibitively expensive and impractical for the average cosmetic practitioner who does not have access to this type of facility.

INJECTION TECHNIQUES

One of the elements of fat grafting technique that is generally agreed on is that engrafted fat survives only when it receives an adequate blood supply from the recipient site.[25] Most investigators also concur that fat cells that are more than 2 mm away from an available vascular source will not survive. Most injection techniques are predicated on the notion that they provide maximal contact between the grafted fat and the host blood supply. In addition, an atraumatic injection technique minimizes damage to the recipient blood supply. Of course, the atraumatic technique also minimizes damage to the adipocytes.

It is inherent to the injection technique that small volumes are injected over multiple small passes through the soft tissue (**Fig. 5**). The techniques differ in the hardware used and the substrate that the fat is injected into. Most investigators place the fat in a series of small tunnels that are at the superficial, mid, and deep layers of the subcutaneous fat. The anatomic basis for this practice is rooted in the goal of keeping each adipocyte as close as possible to the recipient vasculature. In contrast to this practice,[26] there are proponents of injecting the fat directly into the facial musculature. The researchers suggest that this procedure has several benefits. The first is

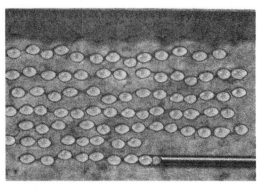

Fig. 5. Small-injection technique.

a diminished amount of periprocedure edema because of the deeper nature of the injection. A more convincing argument is the potentially greater amount of recipient vessels located in the facial muscles. No definitive study has shown this technique to be superior to the standard. Another argument against this technique is the surgeon's desire to recapitulate the natural anatomy of the face. Clearly, the facial fat exists in a plane above the facial muscle, and repeated contraction of the facial muscles might lead to injury and loss of the fat cells. Nonetheless, combining techniques and using intramuscular injection as a component of overall facial rejuvenation must be considered.

Hardware differences are unconvincing as a key element of the technique. Most researchers adhere to the original elements described by Coleman,[27] that is, the use of a blunt-tipped, narrow-gauge injection cannula. There are a wide variety of techniques that diverge from this original configuration. They involve the use of various sizes[28] and tip shapes.[29] There are no significant data to prove that a particular configuration is superior to another. The author uses a variety of small-gauge, blunt-tipped injectors, with the location of treatment being the main determinant of the cannula chosen. A fine-gauge cannula is useful in the periocular region, and a slightly larger cannula is useful in the remainder of the face.

Another interesting study[30] analyzed the role of fat grafting in the restoration of facial contour deformities (volumes) in traumatic and malformation cases. Outcomes were evaluated for each facial aesthetic subunit treated to investigate the role of the recipient site. The study involved 100 patients treated by structural fat grafting of the facial region. Results were evaluated by a subjective self-evaluation survey (ie, a questionnaire answered by patients) and an objective assessment by a 5-member jury. Each subunit of the face was studied separately. The results were significantly different depending on the aesthetic subunit of the face. The best results were achieved in the malar and lateral cheek areas. The poorest results were registered for the lower and upper lip areas. Because the end point of all facial cosmetic procedures is patient satisfaction, it is critical to recognize what areas of the face are well served by fat grafting in the patient's own view.

COMPLICATIONS FROM FAT INJECTION

The injection of autologous fat is considered a safe procedure by most practitioners. Certainly, the technique carries much less risk compared with surgical intervention. There are, however, risks associated with the procedure. Besides the commonplace risks, such as bleeding, infection, bruising, and swelling, there are more major complications. One reported complication is hypertrophy of the engrafted fat. This complication would seem to be contradictory, given the difficulty of getting the fat to survive in the first place. However, episodes of true hypertrophy are reported.[31] Especially concerning about these reports is the time interval between the procedure and complication. In the study cited previously, the complication of hypertrophy was seen as a new complication up to 10 years after the original procedure. More severe complications have been reported, such as the incidence of fat emboli.[32] These complications have been reported to result in significant cerebral injury, such as aphasia and blindness. Although these events are rare, it is important to acknowledge the possibility of these events and include them in the informed consent process.

LOOKING TOWARD THE FUTURE

The area of greatest excitement for autologous fat grafting is the possibility of stem cell treatments. It is well known that harvested fat contains adipose-derived stem cells. There are a variety of protocols that aim to increase the amount of stem cells that are available for reinjection.[33] The effect of stem cell implantation remains unclear. Furthermore, it is difficult to determine the specific action of the stem cell layer of the harvested fat or the fat cells themselves.

There are some elements of facial fat grafting that are hard to explain simply by having a long-term increase in the facial volume. There are descriptions of skin changes that are volume independent and seem to relate to physiologic, rather than structural, changes in the skin. These cases show continued benefit to the facial skin long after the treatments have been completed. This benefit points to an ongoing process that affects the health and biology of the facial skin.[34] Another example of the transformative properties of fat grafting is seen with acne scars. There are good clinical series that show dramatic improvement in the deep atrophic scars associated with acne.[35] Injection of a small amount of fat should do very little to the deep dermal appendages that are associated with these scars. The level of change, therefore, is more consistent with a root change in the local skin biology. As these possible links to stem cell biology become more solidified, there will be a strong impetus to better elucidate the mechanism behind them. Any technique that resupplies facial volume and has long-term positive changes for the appearance of the facial skin will be immensely popular.

REFERENCES

1. Kaufman MR, Miller TA, Huang C, et al. Autologous fat transfer for facial recontouring: is there science behind the art? Plast Reconstr Surg 2007;119:2287–96.
2. Maas CS. Botulinum neurotoxins and injectable fillers: minimally invasive management of the aging upper face. Facial Plast Surg Clin N Am 2007;15(1): 41–9, vi.
3. Scarborough D, Schuen W, Bissaccia E. Fat transfer for aging skin: technique for rhytids. J Dermatol Surg Oncol 1990;16:7.
4. Abbas O, Salman S, Kibbi AG, et al. Localized involutional lipoatrophy with epidermal and dermal changes. J Am Acad Dermatol 2008;58(3):490–3.
5. Hammond E, McKinnon E, Nolan D. Human immunodeficiency virus treatment-induced adipose tissue pathology and lipoatrophy: prevalence and metabolic consequences. Clin Infect Dis 2010;51(5):591–9.
6. Neuber F. Fetttransplantation. Zentrabl Chir 1893;22:66.

7. Miller CG. Cannula implants and review of implantation techniques in esthetic surgery. Chicago: Oak Press; 1926.
8. Axenfeld R. [Uber plastischen Verschluss der Orbita und uber Fetttransplantation zur Beseitgung adharenter Knochennarben am Orbitalrand]. Klin Monatsbl Augenheilkd 1903;41:477 [in German].
9. Marchand F. [Ueber die Veranderungen des Fettgewebes nach der Transplantation]. Beitr Pathol Anat Allg Pathol 1919;66:32 [in German].
10. Peer LA. The neglected free fat graft. Plast Reconstr Surg 1956;18:233.
11. Monheit GD, Prather CL. Juvéderm: a hyaluronic acid dermal filler. J Drugs Dermatol 2007;6(11):1091–5.
12. Coleman SR. Facial recontouring with lipostructure. Clin Plast Surg 1997;24:347.
13. Kaufman MR, Bradley JP, Dickinson B, et al. Autologous fat transfer consensus survey: trends in techniques for harvest, preparation, and application, and perception of short- and long-term results. Plast Reconstr Surg 2007;119:323.
14. Rohrich RJ, Sorokin ES, Brown SA. In search of improved fat transfer viability: a quantitative analysis of the role of centrifugation and harvest site. Plast Reconstr Surg 2004;113:391.
15. Nguyen A, Pasyk KA, Bouvier TN, et al. Comparative study of survival of autologous adipose tissue taken and transplanted by different techniques. Plast Reconstr Surg 1990;85:378.
16. Fagrell D, Enestrom S, Berggren A, et al. Fat cylinder transplantation: an experimental comparative study of three different kinds of fat transplants. Plast Reconstr Surg 1996;98:90.
17. Choo PH, Carter SR, Seiff SR. Lower eyelid volume augmentation with fat pearl grafting. Plast Reconstr Surg 1998;102(5):1716–9.
18. Billings E Jr, May J Jr. Historical review and present status of free fat graft autotransplantation in plastic and reconstructive surgery. Plast Reconstr Surg 1989; 83:368–81.
19. Lidagoster MI, Cinelli PB, Levee EM, et al. Comparison of autologous fat transfer in fresh, refrigerated, and frozen specimens: an animal model. Ann Plast Surg 2000;44:512–5.
20. Wolter TP, Heimburg DV, Stoffels I, et al. Cryopreservation of mature human adipocytes: in vitro measurement of viability. Ann Plast Surg 2005;55:408–13.
21. Pu LL, Coleman SR, Cui X, et al. Cryopreservation of autologous fat grafts harvested with the Coleman technique. Ann Plast Surg 2010;64(3):333–7.
22. Piasecki J, Gutowski K, Lahvis G, et al. An experimental model for improving fat graft viability and purity. Plast Reconstr Surg 2007;119:1571.
23. Yuksel E, Weinfeld A, Cleek R, et al. Increased free fat-graft survival with the long-term, local delivery of insulin, insulin-like growth factor-I, and basic fibroblast growth factor by PLGA/PEG microspheres. Plast Reconstr Surg 2000;105:1712.
24. Shoshani O, Ullmann Y, Shupak A, et al. The role of frozen storage in preserving adipose tissue obtained by suction-assisted lipectomy for repeated fat injection procedures. Dermatol Surg 2001;27:645.
25. Cook T, Nakra T, Shorr N, et al. Facial recontouring with autogenous fat. Facial Plast Surg 2004;20:145.
26. Butterwick KJ, Lack EA. Facial volume restoration with the fat autograft muscle injection technique. Dermatol Surg 2003;29:1019.
27. Coleman SR. Structural fat grafts: the ideal filler? Clin Plast Surg 2001;28:111.
28. Trepsat F. Periorbital rejuvenation combining fat grafting and blepharoplasties. Aesthetic Plast Surg 2003;27:243.

29. Eremia S, Newman N. Long-term follow-up after autologous fat grafting: analysis of results from 116 patients followed at least 12 months after receiving the last of a minimum of two treatments. Dermatol Surg 2000;26:1150.
30. Mojallal A, Shipkov C, Braye F, et al. Influence of the recipient site on the outcomes of fat grafting in facial reconstructive surgery. Plast Reconstr Surg 2009;124(2):471–83.
31. Miller JJ, Popp JC. Fat hypertrophy after autologous fat transfer. Ophthal Plast Reconstr Surg 2002;18(3):228–31.
32. Feinendegen DL, Baumgartner RW, Vuadens P, et al. Autologous fat injection for soft tissue augmentation in the face: a safe procedure? Aesthetic Plast Surg 1998;22:163.
33. Mizuno H, Hyakusoku H. Fat grafting to the breast and adipose-derived stem cells: recent scientific consensus and controversy. Aesthet Surg J 2010;30(3): 381–7.
34. Condé-Green A, de Amorim NF, Pitanguy I. Influence of decantation, washing and centrifugation on adipocyte and mesenchymal stem cell content of aspirated adipose tissue: a comparative study. J Plast Reconstr Aesthet Surg 2010;63(8): 1375–81.
35. Coleman SR. Structural fat grafting: more than a permanent filler. Plast Reconstr Surg 2006;118(Suppl 3):108S–20S.

Breast Augmentation

Marco A. Pelosi III, MD, FICS[a,b,c,d,e,*],
Marco A. Pelosi II, MD, FICS[b,c,d,e]

KEYWORDS

- Breast • Augmentation • Implants • Aesthetic • Cosmetic
- Saline • Silicone • Fat

Breast augmentation is the most commonly performed cosmetic procedure among American women.[1] There are presently 5 ways to augment the breasts in the United States: saline implants, silicone implants, autologous fat injections, external tissue expanders, and tissue flaps. Implants comprise most cosmetic requests, but fat injections are gaining popularity among patients undergoing concomitant liposuction. External tissue expanders are effective for small-volume augmentation, but are not widely used because they are cumbersome and produce variable results. Tissue flaps are a mainstay of reconstructive surgery, but are occasionally used in selected aesthetic cases. The direct injection of synthetic materials into the breast for the purpose of augmentation is not presently approved by the Food and Drug Administration (FDA).

HISTORY

Czerny,[2] credited with the first breast augmentation in 1895, transplanted a lipoma from a woman's back to her chest wall following a mastectomy for benign disease. Gersuny[3] introduced paraffin wax injections for breast, face, and body augmentations in 1900, but subsequently abandoned them because of frequent granulomas, migration, and infections. Liquid silicone breast injections originated as an illicit practice among prostitutes in post-World War II Japan using stolen aircraft fluids.[4] Even after medical-grade silicones became available, continued illicit use, improper medical use, and a tendency to migrate led to many complications and, consequently, this application was made illegal in certain locales. From the late 1940s to the early 1960s, synthetic sponges made from a variety of plastic polymers were tried, but demonstrated numerous problems.[5]

The modern breast implant device was introduced in 1962 by Cronin and Gerow in conjunction with the Dow Corning company.[6] The first-generation silicone prosthesis

The authors have nothing to disclose.

[a] Obstetrics & Gynecology, International College of Surgeons-United States Section, Chicago, IL, USA
[b] American Academy of Cosmetic Surgery, Chicago, IL, USA
[c] American Society of Liposuction Surgery, Chicago, IL, USA
[d] International Society of Cosmetogynecology, Bayonne, NJ, USA
[e] Pelosi Medical Center, 350 Kennedy Boulevard, Bayonne, NJ 07002, USA
* Corresponding author. Pelosi Medical Center, 350 Kennedy Boulevard, Bayonne, NJ 07002.
E-mail address: mpelosi3@pelosimedicalcenter.com

contained a viscous silicone gel within a thick teardrop-shaped silicone shell with prominent seams and Dacron fixation patches on its posterior surface to promote adherence to the chest wall. These implants had a very high incidence of capsular contracture. Second-generation silicone implants were introduced in the early 1970s with the goals of reducing the risk of capsular contracture and of producing a more natural result. These devices were filled with a softer silicone gel, possessed a smooth thinner shell, were round, and no longer displayed fixation patches. Thinner shells led to a new condition known as "gel bleed" in which components of the silicone gel would diffuse through the shell and generate a sticky film and a persisting problem with capsular contracture.[7] A third generation of silicone implants was introduced in the 1980s featuring a stronger double-layered shell and a thicker silicone gel aimed at reducing "gel bleed."[8] Textured surfaces and more viscous cohesive silicone gel marked the next (fourth) generation of silicone implants, which became available in the mid-1980s.[9] Enhanced cohesive (highly cohesive, form-stable, "gummy bear") silicone gel distinguishes the fifth and latest generation of silicone implants, which were introduced in the mid-1990s and are used extensively worldwide, but are presently in FDA clinical trials.[9] Because of FDA mandate, in brief, silicone breast implants for cosmetic enhancement were not available in the United States from 1992 to 2006.

Saline-filled breast implants were introduced in 1965 in an effort to permit smaller skin incisions by filling the device after insertion.[10] The first of these devices had a fill valve permanently attached to its posterior surface that would be sealed manually by the surgeon with a Teflon plug. It was eventually discontinued because of a very high incidence of spontaneous deflation.[11] Modifications in valve design and a thicker shell introduced in the late 1960s led to an acceptable low deflation rate and entry into the American market. At the present time, all saline implants available in the United States are designed to be filled at surgery; prefilled saline implants exist, but have not been cleared by the FDA.

Breast augmentation with injections of autologous fat harvested by liposuction was first described in the early 1980s.[12] Early enthusiasm worldwide was soon tempered by concern, albeit speculative, that such transplants would confound or delay the radiologic diagnosis of breast cancer.[13] Ongoing critical analysis over recent years has demonstrated, however, that these concerns do not appear to be heightened in comparison with other cosmetic breast procedures and these findings have stimulated a renewed interest in this type of breast augmentation.[14,15] To date, this procedure appears best suited for small-volume augmentation and for cosmetic tissue remodeling around existing synthetic breast implants and frequently requires multiple treatment sessions to achieve a desirable lasting result (**Fig. 1**).

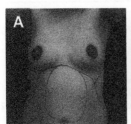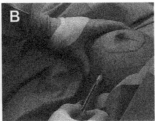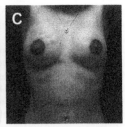

Fig. 1. Breast augmentation with autologous fat. (*A*) Liposuction fat harvest areas are marked. (*B*) Fat is transplanted into the breast with multiple small-volume injections. (*C*) Appearance 1 day after surgery with 200 mL of fat injected into each breast.

Breast augmentation with external tissue expanders was introduced in 1999.[16] The method, currently known as the Brava system, uses a pair of self-sealing rigid polyurethane domes that are applied directly over the breasts to create a negative pressure that causes tissue distraction, which, in turn, stimulates tissue growth (**Fig. 2**). Although the technology is effective, it has not gained popularity because it requires a minimum of 10 hours of continuous daily use for a minimum of 10 weeks to produce results, and the results, under the best of circumstances, are typically less than a 1-cup-size augmentation.

PATIENT SELECTION AND ASSESSMENT

The best candidates for breast augmentation with implants are nonobese women displaying relatively symmetric breasts, a symmetric frame, and lacking breast ptosis (**Fig. 3**). Ptosis is evaluated with the patient standing and is defined as descent of the center of the nipple-areola complex (NAC) below the level of the inframammary fold (IMF) and is commonly graded as mild (0 to 1-cm descent), moderate (1- to 3-cm descent), or severe (>3-cm descent). Subcategories and alternate classification systems have been proposed primarily for the design of mastopexy (breast-lifting) procedures rather than for augmentation and are not addressed herein. The tissues into which the implants are to be placed are referred to as the tissue envelope and the characteristics of the envelope define both the implant dimensions and tissue planes best suited for the individual patient.

A complete documented medical evaluation including appropriate screening for preexisting breast disease and risk factors should precede any cosmetic breast surgery. Any anatomic distortion with the potential to increase the risk of injury or asymmetry should be assessed and managed by appropriate means before surgery. Blood work analyses include testing for signs of infection, anemia, coagulopathy, and liver disease. Pregnancy testing is performed or repeated on the day of surgery irrespective of history. If the physician performing the medical evaluation is not the surgeon and is unfamiliar with the proposed operation, basic relevant details of the planned anesthetic agents and surgical interventions should be provided along with the request for medical clearance.

Patients most frequently verbalize their desired goal in terms of brassiere cup size, but do not always have a well-defined concept of their appearance at the requested size. To facilitate the selection process, it is helpful to use a photographic portfolio of women of similar build augmented with implants of various sizes preferably operated

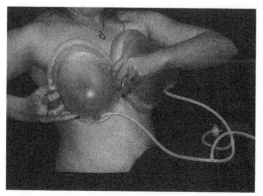

Fig. 2. The Brava external tissue expansion device is being applied. Negative pressure created by a vacuum pump causes tissue distraction, which, in turn, causes tissue growth. Prolonged use is required and augmentation results are modest.

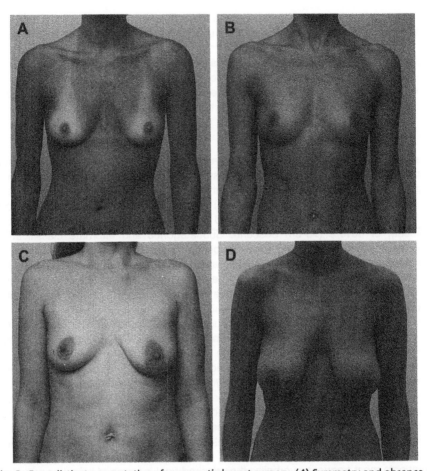

Fig. 3. Four distinct presentations for cosmetic breast surgery. (*A*) Symmetry and absence of ptosis are ideal for implants. (*B*) Slight size asymmetry requires larger implant on left side. (*C*) Unilateral mild ptosis, size asymmetry, and areolar asymmetry warrants unilateral mastopexy and bilateral implants. (*D*) Severe symmetric ptosis warrants bilateral mastopexy without implants.

by the same surgeon. Other aids include sizer implants and sizer brassieres, which permit the surgeon to evaluate the difference in volume between the desired cup size and the existing breast tissue. Computer-generated photographic imaging software is widely marketed, but currently lacks the sophistication necessary to produce realistic images of the many variations of the augmented breast as they relate to the specific tissue planes and the qualities of the native soft tissue coverage. The visualization process is further enhanced by having the patient spend a few days wearing sizer implants at her desired size in different styles of clothing. The counseling process should include a discussion about the degree of attention that the requested size may generate as well as the physical consequences that the implants may have on the body, especially if the request reaches or exceeds the limits of the soft tissue coverage. In general, the larger the implant, the greater the risk for unfavorable cosmetic outcomes.

Medications, supplements, herbs, and other substances with the capacity to impair coagulation should be discontinued in advance of surgery. Substances that interact negatively with anesthetic agents and perioperative medications should also be with-held. If they cannot be discontinued or substituted, the surgical plan will need to be modified, delayed, or withheld. Cigarette smoking is not a contraindication to breast augmentation, but smokers typically display a higher incidence of capsular contrac-tion and rippling than nonsmokers and must be counseled appropriately.

Expectations and motivations need to be explored in depth when addressing the cosmetic patient. Unrealistic expectations will never be fulfilled by surgery even if executed to perfection by any medical or aesthetic standard. The cosmetic surgery "addict," the "perfectionist," and the patient expecting cosmetic surgery to remedy interpersonal conflicts are examples of misguided personality types to be screened out at the initial consultation.

ANESTHESIA

Breast implants may be placed under local anesthesia with or without intravenous sedation or general anesthesia. Each modality has its advantages, disadvantages, inherent risks, and suitability for the unique demands of each operation and patient. Regardless of technique, the surgical team should be knowledgeable and prepared and the facility should be equipped to manage all potential adverse drug effects.

ANATOMY

Embryologically, the breast bud develops into the breast gland within Scarpa fascia, splitting it into an anterior and a posterior layer (lamellae) which are commonly termed the superficial and deep layers of superficial fascia, respectively. These lamellae remain connected to one another via fibers known as Cooper ligaments, which provide support to the breast. The posterior lamella of the breast rests primarily on the fascia of the pectoralis major muscle and to a much lesser extent on the fascia of surrounding muscles (serratus anterior, external oblique, rectus abdominis).

The vascular supply to the breast is diffuse. The main supply derives from the internal mammary artery (internal thoracic artery) via perforators through the medial chest wall and the lateral intercostal perforators, which derive from the lateral thoracic artery. Superiorly, the breast is supplied by the thoracoacromial artery perforators. The venous drainage system closely follows the arterial supply. The lymphatic system is not disrupted to any significant degree by breast augmentation procedures.

INCISION SITES AND IMPLANT POCKETS

The 3 main decisions made in any breast augmentation are implant selection, incision site, and tissue plane (pocket plane). For a given patient, there are frequently a variety of acceptable approaches to reach the desired goal. Common incision sites include the inframammary fold, the periareolar region, and the axilla. Other options include the umbilicus and through the upper margin of an abdominoplasty flap. There are 4 possible pocket planes for implant insertion: the subglandular plane, the subpectoral or partial submuscular plane, the subfascial plane above the pectoralis major muscle, and the total submuscular plane.

The inframammary incision was the original approach to breast implant insertion and it remains popular among surgeons because it provides the most direct route of implant insertion, excellent exposure, and the greatest ability to expand the incision as needed. All 4 pocket planes can be accessed via the inframammary route. For certain types of larger prefilled devices, such as form-stable highly cohesive silicone gel implants, this may be the only viable approach that avoids damage to either surrounding structures or to the prosthesis itself in the process of insertion. Nonetheless, this approach inevitably leaves a visible scar, which detracts from its popularity among women especially those in whom less than ideal scarring and keloid formation are of concern. Important technical aspects of the inframammary incision include a location slightly lateral to the midline to permit easy access to the border of the pectoralis major (**Fig. 4**), and the identification and preservation of Scarpa fascia along the natural inframammary fold to support the weight of the implant and avoid a bottoming out of the prosthesis over time.

The periareolar approach is technically easy, permits a rapid pocket dissection in any of the 4 pocket planes, and typically leaves an indistinct scar. Limitations include the inability to expand the incision in the presence of a small areola for the insertion of a large prefilled implant and the inevitable breach of the breast parenchyma that accompanies the requisite dissection process. Also, exposure may be difficult to generate if the areola is small. This route carries the highest risk of implant infection owing to the proximity of the breast ductal system, colonized with skin-borne bacteria, to the surgical field. This route is favored by many nonendoscopically trained surgeons especially for the subpectoral implant pocket because it provides good direct visualization for muscle division. Keys to an optimal cosmetic result include maintenance of the incision entirely within the border of the pigmented areolar skin, precise reapproximation of the incision edges, and selecting patients with an adequately large areolar diameter.

Transaxillary breast augmentation was originally developed as a blind approach in the early 1970s and evolved into an endoscopic approach in the early 1990s. All 4 pocket planes may be accessed via this route. The axilla scars well even in women prone to hypertrophic scarring because of the lack of skin tension in the area and incisions placed high within the axillary dome cannot be viewed in most positions of the arm (**Fig. 5**). The blind approach has its few stalwart "dying breed" proponents from the nonendoscopic era, but the inability to confirm hemostasis and accurate dissection of the pocket directly cannot be disputed. The endoscopic approach relies on basic techniques, equipment, and skills familiar to any surgeon with training and experience in laparoscopic surgery. Because of the magnified field of view, it affords unparalleled exposure and control of the surgical field and precise dissection. Essential details of the axillary incision include incision placement high within a skin crease in the axillary dome behind the lateral border of the pectoralis major to minimize scar

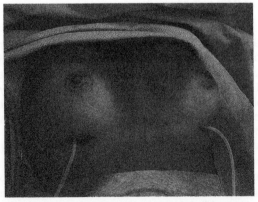

Fig. 4. Inframammary incision for subpectoral implants is made slightly lateral off-center from nipple to permit better access to lateral border of pectoralis major muscle.

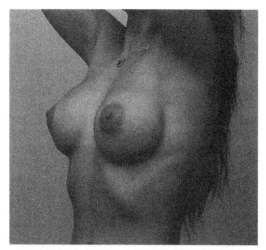

Fig. 5. The axillary incision placed high in the dome of the axilla along a natural skin crease is indistinct 1 year after surgery.

visibility and subcutaneous dissection around the intercostobrachial nerve, which provides sensory innervation along the posteriomedial upper arm (**Fig. 6**).

Transumbilical breast augmentation (TUBA) was developed in the early 1990s based on concepts and techniques derived from breast implant insertion via abdominoplasty flap dissections. The technique relies on the dissection of bilateral access

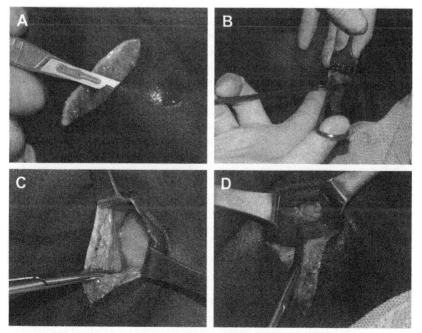

Fig. 6. Key steps of the axillary incision protect the intercostobrachial nerve, which crosses perpendicular to the skin incision in the superficial fat. (*A*) Undermining of skin from fat. (*B*) Superficial tunneling anterior to the nerve. (*C*) Atraumatic retraction of nerve and fat to expose pectoralis major fascia. (*D*) Lateral border of pectoralis major muscle exposed.

tunnels from the umbilicus to the inframammary fold by palpation using a large blunt-tipped tube and blunt development of the implant pocket with long dissectors and an expander. Only the subglandular and subpectoral pockets can be accessed by current methods. TUBA is a blind approach, but an endoscope is frequently used to verify the subpectoral plane and to confirm hemostasis. Bleeding and hematomas are less common with TUBA than with other techniques, but conversion to another incision is necessary if hemostatic control cannot be achieved by other means. The nature of the access tunnels limits this operation to inflatable saline implants.

The subglandular (prepectoral) pocket is made in the loose areolar tissue plane that exists between the deep superficial fascia of the breast envelope (posterior lamella) and the fascia overlying the pectoralis major and serratus anterior muscles. This pocket is generally acceptable for women with adequate subcutaneous tissue thickness in the upper pole of the breast to provide adequate coverage of the upper half of the breast implant. It is also frequently used when augmenting a slightly ptotic breast because it permits the lax tissues to spread evenly without clinging to the pectoralis fascia. The dissection is relatively simple and postoperative discomfort is minimal because muscle dissection is not required. Subglandular implants carry a higher risk of rippling around their periphery because the plane is close to the skin. They also carry a higher risk of capsular contracture than implants placed beneath the pectoralis muscles.

The subpectoral (partial submuscular, dual-plane, biplanar) pocket is created immediately beneath the pectoralis major muscle and above the rib cage and pectoralis minor muscle. Adequate dissection of the implant space warrants full-thickness division of the pectoralis major fibers along the inferior margin of the breast and blunt mobilization of the serratus anterior muscle along the lateral margin of the pocket. Division of the pectoralis major fibers creates a gap in the muscle that exposes the overlying breast tissue to the implant in the lower pole of the breast (subglandular plane) while muscle tissue remains to cover the implant in the upper pole of the breast (submuscular plane). Patients do not experience a loss of arm strength or function from this type of muscle division because most of the pectoralis major muscle remains intact along its medial and superior attachments to the chest wall. The subpectoral pocket is favored for women with minimal subcutaneous tissue in the upper pole of the breast. It also carries the lowest risk of capsular contracture presumably owing to the constant motion of the breast implant in response to the regular action of the overlying muscle. Subpectoral implants have a tendency to distort the contour of the breast to varying degrees when the pectoralis major muscle contracts. This is not a major issue for most women, but is of concern to female body builders in particular.

The subfascial pocket, a potential space between the pectoralis major and serratus muscles and their overlying fascia, was first described in the late 1990s, initially via the axillary approach and subsequently via the periareolar and inframammary routes.[17] Characteristics of the space are similar to those of the traditional subglandular pocket, but it offers slightly more tissue coverage at the implant edges and offers another option to women who will not tolerate implant distortion related to pectoralis muscle contraction.

The total submuscular pocket is essentially a subpectoral pocket without any division of the pectoralis major fibers along the lower pole of the breast along with partial mobilization of the serratus anterior muscle fibers along the inferolateral pocket margin. The only advantage to this space is decreased palpability of the inferior border of the implant in the presence of minimal native tissue thickness along the inframammary fold. Dissection of the serratus anterior fibers is not along any natural plane and implants placed in this pocket have a tendency to ride high (superior malposition) over time. This is the least commonly used pocket.

When the breast is augmented with autologous fat injections, the fat is layered throughout the periphery of the breast tissue rather than directly into the center of the stroma. It is sometimes also injected into the pectoralis major muscle. To maximize the surface area of injected fat in contact with an adequate blood supply in the recipient tissues, it is transplanted with multiple small-volume passes rather than with large-volume depot injections. Injection sites are commonly placed at the areolar border, the inframammary fold, and the axillary fold. The recipient sites are frequently injected with vasoconstrictive solutions to minimize bruising and to reduce the risk of intravascular injection; blunt-tipped needles are used exclusively.

PERIOPERATIVE CONSIDERATIONS

All techniques of breast augmentation begin with systematic and precise markings of the proposed pocket margins, incision sites, and anatomic landmarks, preferably in the standing position (**Fig. 7**). Volume asymmetry is carefully assessed, as are the thickness of the tissue envelope in the upper and lower poles of the breast, and the distance from the nipple to the inframammary fold. Measurements are recorded and markings are photographed.

Antibiotic prophylaxis before and after surgery is mandatory when implanting a prosthetic device and should target common pathogens of the skin and breast ductal system. Spare implants should be available in case the primary implants are damaged or contaminated; they should remain available in the immediate postoperative phase in the event that unexpected findings warrant explantation, revision, and replantation. If the surgeon wishes to have some flexibility in the choice of implants, a variety of sizes should be stocked. Implant makers provide consignment arrangements that make it relatively simple to maintain an array of different models and sizes.

The surgical suite should be equipped with an operating table that can flex the patient from supine to upright to assess final implant position. Noninvasive monitoring of blood pressure, electrocardiogram, and pulse oximetry should not encroach upon the surgical field. The skin is cleansed thoroughly with betadine or similar agents. Some surgeons prefer to cover the nipple-areola complex with an occlusive dressing for the duration of the surgery to minimize bacterial contamination of the surgical field. Frequent and copious irrigation is used, but the ideal solution has yet to be

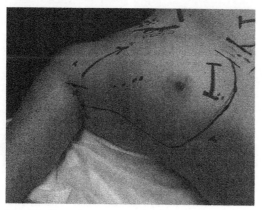

Fig. 7. Surgical markings indicate base anatomic dimensions, the margins of the implant pocket, incision location, and anatomic landmarks.

established. The most common irrigants are either dilute antibiotic mixtures or diluted betadine. Specialized blunt dissectors are commonly used to expand and shape the implant pocket (**Fig. 8**). Surgical drains are used when deemed necessary, but prolonged use may increase the risk of infection.

After surgery, absorbent dressings are placed over all incision sites and elastic stabilization bands are applied above and sometimes below the implants. For subpectoral implants, muscle relaxants aid in reducing postoperative discomfort especially for reflex tension of the back muscles. Most patients describe varying degrees of pressure over the chest from the implants, which increases with inspiration through the first day after surgery. General discomfort is proportional to implant size and is managed with either oral narcotic or nonsteroidal medications. Patients are reassessed for proper healing and band placement on the first day after surgery, then weekly for the first few weeks thereafter. Supportive and underwire-type brassieres are avoided until the implants have settled into proper position—a process that may take several weeks or even months. Until that time, nipple shields or sports bras are used. Patients with subglandular implants are instructed in the performance of breast exercises 2 to 3 times daily beginning in the second postoperative week to help prevent capsular contracture and may resume full activity in 3 weeks. Patients with subpectoral implants do not require breast exercises and are counseled to avoid exercise or vigorous use of the chest muscles for the first 6 weeks after surgery. The ability to turn a steering wheel without pain determines the patient's readiness to resume driving a motor vehicle.

Breast augmentation by autologous fat grafting is performed on the same day as the liposuction harvesting procedure to maximize tissue viability and to minimize the risk for infection. The fat is harvested using narrow-caliber liposuction cannulas to facilitate

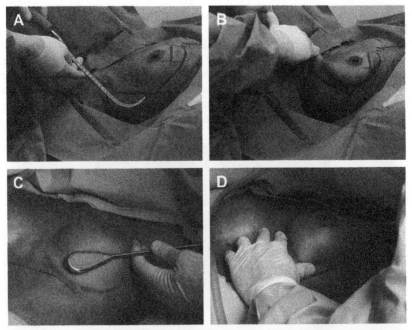

Fig. 8. Common breast dissectors. (*A, B*) Agris-Dingman "hockey stick" blunt dissector is used for general expansion of lateral and inferior implant pocket. (*C, D*) Flat paddle blunt dissector is used for minor pocket adjustments sometimes with implant or sizer in place.

reinjection with narrow-caliber fat transfer cannulas. Low-suction pressures are used to minimize barotrauma to the harvested fat and technologies that destroy adipocytes, such as ultrasound and laser, are avoided. These procedures are commonly performed under local anesthesia and the recipient site is often injected with a lower volume of the same anesthetic solution used for the liposuction procedure. The patient is fitted with a tight conforming surgical bra, which is worn continuously for the first few weeks after surgery. There is some loss of volume over time, but the final breast shape typically stabilizes by the sixth month. The need for additional fat-grafting sessions is common.

COMPLICATIONS

Complications of breast augmentation with either implants or fat may relate directly to the surgical procedure itself, to the immediate cosmetic outcome, to delayed long-term changes of the augmented breast, or to the prosthesis. Some cosmetic changes may be viewed either positively or negatively depending on the patient's expectations.

Bleeding-related problems may arise intraoperatively upon intended or unintended division of any of the high-pressure intercostal and internal mammary perforator blood vessels that course along the lateral and medial borders of the implant pocket at various levels of dissection. Control is straightforward provided the surgical field is well exposed, but delayed bleeding may result in hematoma formation. In the hypertensive patient, low-level oozing may be seen despite careful dissection and management may include the placement of temporary surgical drains. Although implants provide a degree of tamponnade, this effect should not be relied on as a substitute for hemostatic surgical technique. Blood left within the pocket may provoke significant discomfort and increase the risks for infection and capsular contracture. Hematomas of the implant pocket typically produce swelling, bruising, and extreme discomfort of the affected breast and warrant prompt surgical exploration. Seromas or delayed hematomas produce painless swelling and firmness of the breast, are not associated with bruising, and are treated with surgical drainage with or without implant exchange; sonography is a useful diagnostic aid.

Infection may complicate breast implant surgery at the external incision site or around the prosthesis itself. Incisional infections not involving the implant are treated with antibiotics and evacuation of any localized pus if present. Infections involving the implant warrant immediate bilateral explantation, antibiotic therapy, and a delay of replantation of several months. Delayed surgical intervention increases the risk for permanent disfigurement of the breast.

Damage to the integrity of the chest wall is a risk of any operation in the thoracic region and fortunately is not common with breast augmentation. Pneumothorax has been reported to occur with breast augmentations performed under both local and general anesthesia and has been diagnosed intra- and postoperatively. Various mechanisms of injury have been either identified or postulated to include pleural lacerations during dissection, needle puncture of the pleura with injection of local anesthetics, rupture of pulmonary blebs or bullae related to high anesthetic ventilation pressures, and barotrauma in cases where large implants are forcibly inserted through small incisions into pockets with trapped air.[18]

Capsular contracture is the most common complication of breast implant surgery and the risk is highest with silicone implants. The etiology is unknown, but is thought to be inflammatory and related to bacterial contamination.[19] The Baker grading system is commonly used to describe the degree of contracture with Grade I defined as the normal, soft breast texture; Grade II is a firm breast texture with normal contours; Grade III is a firm breast texture with altered breast contours; and becomes

Grade IV if the breast is painful as a result of the condition. Treatment is reserved for Grades III and IV only and involves total or partial capsulectomy depending on the risk of chest wall injury with dissection of deep, adherent capsules. The prevention of this condition drives many surgical protocols and implant design modifications and is an area of intense ongoing research.

Asymmetry relating to breast volume or contour or inframammary fold level may exist either before or after surgery (**Fig. 9**). The nipple-areola complex may vary significantly between both breasts and ptosis may be unilateral. Preoperative asymmetries must be pointed out at the initial consultation and variations in the surgical plan and choice of implants carefully and thoroughly discussed so that the patient understands the limitations of each step in the process, especially if the achievement of relative symmetry will require additional incisions. Postoperative asymmetries may affect any aspect of the breast contour as well as the level of the inframammary fold and some may require surgical revision of the pocket, whereas others may require repositioning of the nipple-areola complex.

Wrinkling and rippling of the tissues along the edges of the implant is sometimes seen, especially with large implants placed into small breasts where the tissue envelope is prone to thinning over time. No singular cause for rippling has been identified, but it is more commonly seen with textured saline implants, subglandular pockets, and cigarette smokers. Management options include replacing affected saline implants with silicone implants or targeting the ripples directly with injections of autologous fat.

Synmastia is a rare complication of breast implant surgery in which the implant pockets fuse across the midline resulting in a loss of cleavage. It is thought to result from aggressive medial dissection or excessively large implants.[20] Correction involves positioning implants in an alternate pocket and suturing the medial borders of the existing defects. Preventive measures include the avoidance of dissection close to the midline and preservation of the medial pectoralis fibers when placing subpectoral implants.

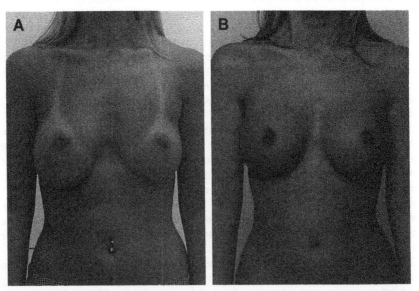

Fig. 9. (A) Presentation 17 months post inframammary subpectoral saline augmentation with acute deflation of left implant and inferior malposition "bottoming out" of right implant. (B) Treatment consisted of elevation of right inframammary fold and replacement of both implants via inframammary incisions and was performed under local anesthesia.

Device failure may present as deflation of a saline implant or rupture of a silicone implant. Saline implants may deflate as a result of valve failure, chronic creasing of the shell if underfilled, or trauma. Failure generates a rapid and obvious loss of volume as the saline is rapidly absorbed (see **Fig. 9**). Silicone implant rupture does not result in loss of volume and thus, may be unknown to the patient. Most ruptured silicone implants are diagnosed at the time of revisionary surgery for unrelated reasons and in most, the silicone is contained within the biologic capsule. Magnetic resonance imaging is advocated as the modality of choice for screening for implant rupture, but patients with claustrophobia or certain types of implanted hardware are not candidates and different generations of silicone implants demonstrate different radiologic characteristics of rupture.[21]

Breast cancer is not a complication of breast augmentation by any modality, but the augmented breast complicates standard mammographic screening.[22] Mammographic displacement studies and magnetic resonance imaging are frequently used to better assess areas that are obscured by implants on routine mammographic views. Tumors of the breast parenchyma are typically easier to palpate in the presence of implants and can be biopsied by standard open techniques, but deeper lesions may require temporary removal of the implant for access.[23] Although studies are limited, breast implants do not appear to affect breast cancer survival.[22]

Changes resulting from autologous fat injections to the breast may include palpable lumps, fat necrosis, liponecrotic cysts, and calcifications that are distinct from those of malignancy.[14] None of these changes are unique to fat transfer and may occur with any type of breast surgery including breast reduction, breast biopsy, reconstructive procedures, implants, radiation therapy, and liposuction.[14] The most common undesirable outcome of breast augmentation with transplanted fat is a partial loss of the implanted volume, which has been reported to range from 30% to 60% of the original volume in sonographic studies.[24]

SUMMARY

Breast augmentation is the most commonly performed cosmetic procedure among American women. Saline implants, silicone implants, and autologous fat injections are the most common options. The inframammary, periareolar, and axillary approaches with or without endoscopy are the most common routes of implantation. The subpectoral dual-plane and the subglandular plane are the most common pockets. The most common complications are capsular contracture for implants and volume loss for injected fat. Breast augmentation does not appear to increase breast cancer risk or survival rates.

REFERENCES

1. Cosmetic Surgery National Data Bank. 2008 Statistics. New York (NY): American Society for Aesthetic Plastic Surgery; 2009. p. 3.
2. Czerny V. Plastischer ersatz der brustdrüse durch ein lipom. Zentralbl Chir 1895; 22:72 [in German].
3. Gersuny R. [Uber eine subcutane prosthes.] Zeitschrift Heikunde Wien u Leipzig 1900;21:199 [in German].
4. Chasan PE. The history of injectable silicone fluids for soft-tissue augmentation. Plast Reconstr Surg 2007;120:2034–40.
5. Spear SL, Parikh PM, Goldstein JA. History of breast implants and the Food and Drug Administration. Clin Plast Surg 2009;36:15–21.

6. Cronin TD, Gerow FJ. Augmentation mammoplasty: a new "natural feel" prosthesis. Transactions of the Third International Congress of plastic surgery. Amsterdam (The Netherlands): Excerpta Medica Foundation; 1964. p. 41–9.
7. Barker DE, Retsky MI, Schultz S. "Bleeding" of silicone from bag-gel breast implants and its clinical relation to fibrous capsule reaction. Plast Reconstr Surg 1978;61:836–41.
8. Price JE, Barker DE. Initial clinical experience with low bleed breast implants. Aesthetic Plast Surg 1983;7:255–6.
9. Maxwell GP, Gabriel A. The evolution of breast implants. Clin Plast Surg 2009;36: 1–13.
10. Arion HG. Retromammary prosthesis. C R Soc Fr Gynecol 1965;35:427.
11. Williams JE. Experiences with a large series of silastic breast implants. Plast Reconstr Surg 1972;49:253–8.
12. Bircoll MJ. Case report: cosmetic breast augmentation utilizing autologous fat and liposuction techniques. Plast Reconstr Surg 1987;79:267–71.
13. ASPRS Ad-Hoc Committee on New Procedures. Report on autologous fat transplantation. Plast Surg Nurs Winter 1987;7(4):140–1.
14. Coleman SR, Saboeiro AP. Fat grafting to the breast revisited: safety and efficacy. Plast Reconstr Surg 2007;119:775–85.
15. Gutowski KA. Current applications and safety of autologous fat grafts: a report of the ASPS Fat Graft Task Force. Plast Reconstr Surg 2009;124:272–80.
16. Khoury RK, Schlenz I, Murphy BJ, et al. Nonsurgical breast enlargement using an external soft-tissue expansion system. Plast Reconstr Surg 2000;105:2500–12.
17. Graf RM, Bernardes A, Auersvald A, et al. Subfascial endoscopic transaxillary augmentation mammaplasty. Aesthetic Plast Surg 2000;24:216–20.
18. Fayman MS. Air drainage: an essential technique for preventing breast augmentation-related pneumothorax. Aesthetic Plast Surg 2007;31:19–22.
19. Adams WP. Capsular contracture: what is it? What causes it? How can it be prevented and managed. Clin Plast Surg 2009;36:119–26.
20. Spear SL, Bogue DP, Thomassen JM. Synmastia after breast augmentation. Plast Reconstr Surg 2006;118(Suppl):168S–71S.
21. Gorczyca DP, Gorczyca SM, Gorczyca KL. The diagnosis of silicone breast implant rupture. Plast Reconstr Surg 2007;120(No. 7, Suppl 1):49S–61S.
22. Deapen D. Breast implants and breast cancer: a review of incidence, detection, mortality, and survival. Plast Reconstr Surg 2007;120(No. 7, Suppl 1):70S–80S.
23. Nahabedian MY, Patel K. Management of common and uncommon problems after primary breast augmentation. Clin Plast Surg 2009;36:127–38.
24. Wang H, Jiang Y, Yu Y, et al. Sonographic assessment on breast augmentation after autologous fat graft. Plast Reconstr Surg 2008;122(No. 1):36e–8e.

Cosmeceuticals: Practical Applications

Anetta E. Reszko, MD, PhD[a],*, Diane Berson, MD[a,b],
Mary P. Lupo, MD[c]

KEYWORDS

- Antioxidants • Cosmeceuticals • Procedure protocols
- Vitamins • Pigment-lightening • Anti-inflammatory • Peptides

Cosmeceutical is a term coined approximately 2 decades ago by Albert Kligman to refer to topically applied products that are not merely cosmetics that adorn or camouflage, yet are not true drugs that have undergone rigorous placebo-controlled studies for safety and efficacy.[1] This continues to be an area of new product development, with an ever-growing marketplace as baby boomers continue to age. There are many review articles that outline the theoretical biologic and clinical actions of these cosmeceuticals and their various ingredients.[2–7] This article reviews how to incorporate various cosmeceuticals into the treatment regime of patients, depending on the diagnosis and treatment chosen. The practical application of when, why, and on whom to use different products will enable physicians to improve the methodology of product selection and, ultimately, improve patient's clinical results.

Cosmeceuticals can be divided into 7 main product categories (**Box 1**).

In choosing an effective cosmeceuticals regimen it is critical to match patients and their problems with the appropriate products. Most patients have multiple needs, and

This article originally appeared in *Dermatologic Clinics* 2009;27(4):401–416.
[a] Department of Dermatology, Weill Cornell Medical College of Cornell University, 1305 York Avenue, 9th Floor, New York, New York 10021, USA
[b] Private Practice, 211 East 53 Street, New York, New York 10022, USA
[c] Department of Dermatology, Tulane Medical School, Private Practice Lupo Center for Aesthetic and General Dermatology, 145 Robert E Lee Boulevard, Suite 302, New Orleans, LA 70124, USA
* Corresponding author.
E-mail address: anetta.reszko@gmail.com

Obstet Gynecol Clin N Am 37 (2010) 547–569
doi:10.1016/j.ogc.2010.09.006
0889-8545/10/$ – see front matter © 2010 Elsevier Inc. All rights reserved.

Box 1
Cosmeceuticals product categories

- Sunscreen
- Antioxidant
- Anti-inflammatory
- Pigment lightening
- Collagen repair
- Exfoliation
- Hydration/barrier repair

---

they should be matched with products that offer ingredients with multifactorial benefits.

Certain treatment principles apply to all therapeutic protocols. Morning treatment protocols should provide environmental (antioxidant, sunscreen, sun block) and anti-microbial protection whereas evening/night protocols should be centered on tissue repair (retinoid).

This article highlights several common diagnoses and discusses how and which cosmeceuticals should help, or at least compliment, procedures or prescriptions. Furthermore, the use of cosmeceuticals in conjunction with commonly performed office-based procedures, such as chemical peels, microdermabrasion, photorejuvenation, and laser resurfacing, is discussed.

MELASMA
Introduction

Even skin pigmentation is considered to be a universal sign of youth and beauty. Pigmentary alterations seen in melasma are sharply demarcated, brown patches, typically located on the malar prominences and forehead. Three clinically apparent patterns are centrofacial, malar, and mandibular (rare). Melasma is more frequent in higher skin types (III, IV, and V) and is especially prominent among Asian and Hispanic people. The pigment deposition in melasma is epidermally or dermally based, with most cases showing both.

Treatment of melasma is often difficult and might require multiple treatment modalities. Sunlight protection with a broad-spectrum sunscreen with ultraviolet A (UVA) and ultraviolet B (UVB) coverage is the cornerstone of the therapy, because UVB, UVA, and visible light are all capable of stimulating melanogenesis. Sunscreens and sun blockers containing physical blockers, such as titanium dioxide and zinc oxide, are preferable to chemical blockers because of their broader protection.

The mainstay of treatment of melasma is topical depigmenting agents (**Box 2**).

In addition, retinoids, exfoliation with superficial chemical peels, mechanical dermabrasion, or nonablative (intense pulsed light [IPL]) or fractional microablative technologies may provide added benefit. Combination therapy centers on the fact that if melanogenesis is inhibited (depigmenting agents) and keratinocyte turnover is increased (chemical peels, retinoids, lasers/IPL), the time to clinical improvement can be reduced.

Pigment Modifying Agents

Currently available pigment lightening products target individual stages of melanogenesis or block melanin transfer from melanocytes to keratinocytes. The following are commercially available, highly effective pigment lightening preparations.

Box 2
Pigment modifying agents
Hydroquinone
Kojic acid
Vitamins C and E
Azelaic acid
Ellagic acid (polyphenol)
Pycnogenol
Fatty acids (linoloic acid)
Niacinamide (B3)
Soy (STI)

Hydroquinone

Hydroquinone (HQ), benzene-1,4-diol, is an inhibitor of melanogenesis by (1) inhibiting tyrosinase, and (2) a direct melanocyte cytotoxic effect. HQ is a poor substrate of tyrosinase, competing for tyrosine oxidation in active melanocytes. The cytotoxic effect of HQ is mediated by reversible inhibition of DNA and RNA synthesis.

Clinical improvement with over-the-counter 2% HQ as monotherapy is usually seen in 4 to 6 weeks, with improvement approaching a plateau at 4 months. Because of its irritant properties and increased risk of postinflammatory hyperpigmentation (PIH), HQ is often combined with topical medium potency steroids. Compounded HQ is available in the United States as Tri-Luma (Galderma, Fort Worth, TX, USA; 0.01% fluocinolone, 4% HQ and 0.05% tretinoin) in a cream formulation.[5]

In recent years, the use of HQ has become a subject of marked controversy, that led to its removal from markets in Europe and in parts of Asia.[5] In recent months, the Food and Drug Administration (FDA) voiced concerns about the safety of HQ for topical application. The basis for the FDA's concern was the increasing number of reports of ochronosis, (bluish-black discoloration) of HQ topically treated sites,[8] and reports of potential carcinogenicity of systemic HQ. The mechanism of HQ-induced ochronosis remains unknown. It is usually observed in patients of African descent who have been treated with high concentrations of HQ for several years. Histologically, the initial stages of ochronosis are characterized by the degeneration of collagen and elastic fibers. In later stages, ochronotic deposits are seen, consisting of crescent-shaped, ochre-colored fibers in the dermis. It is unclear whether HQ itself, high concentrations of HQ, or other substances that exist in the topical preparations contribute to the onset of ochronosis.

The carcinogenic properties of HQ were demonstrated in rodent models following systemic administration of high quantities of HQ. The human potential for carcinogenicity has not been demonstrated. Nonetheless, because of the rapid uptake and distribution of HQ applied to the skin, it has been speculated that the risks of topical application are similar to, or greater than, those of pulmonary or gastrointestinal exposure.[9] With topical application, the first-pass liver metabolism of HQ is circumvented and HQ, a benzene derivate, can reach systemic circulation without prior detoxification.

Azelaic acid

Azelaic acid is a naturally occurring, saturated 9-carbon dicarboxylic acid derived from *Pityrosporum ovale*. It is a weak competitive inhibitor of tyrosinase. Azelaic acid also exhibits antiproliferative and cytotoxic effects on melanocytes via inhibition of thioredoxin reductase, an enzyme involved in mitochondrial oxidoreductase activation and DNA synthesis. Unlike HQ, azelaic acid seems to target only abnormally hyperactive melanocytes, and thus will not lighten skin with normally functioning melanocytes. Thus, the benefits of azelaic acid might extend beyond the realm of cosmetic medicine, as it may play a role in preventing development of, or in therapy for, lentigo maligna and lentigo maligna melanoma.[5,6]

The clinical efficacy and pigment lightening properties of azelaic acid have been studied in large groups of diverse skin types, including skin types III to VI, and its efficacy has been compared with that of 4% HQ cream, although with a slightly higher rate of local irritation.[10,11] Azelaic acid is commercially available as a topical 20% cream. The primary adverse effect of topical application is skin irritation. For added benefit, azelaic acid may be combined with 15–20% glycolic acid (GA).

Niacinamide

Niacinamide, also known as nicotinamide, is a water-soluble component of the vitamin B complex group. In vivo, nicotinamide is incorporated into nicotinamide adenine dinucleotide (NAD) and nicotinamide adenine dinucleotide phosphate (NADP), coenzymes essential for enzymatic oxidation reduction reactions, including tissue mitochondrial respiration and lipid metabolism.

Niacinamide inhibits melanine transfer to keratinocyte. Bissett and colleagues[12–15] showed that niacinamide reduced the appearance of hyperpigmented macules, fine lines and wrinkles, red blotchiness, skin sallowness, and increased skin elasticity. In addition, niacinamide helped alleviate some of the symptoms of rosacea by increasing hydration, reducing transepidermal water loss, and improving the barrier function of the stratum corneum.

Kojic acid

Kojic acid, 5-hydroxymethyl-4*H*-pyrane-4-one, is a hydrophilic fungal derivative derived from *Aspergillus* and *Penicillium* species, exerting its biologic activity by inhibiting copper binding to tyrosinase. It is one of the most commonly used over-the-counter skin lightening agents sold worldwide. Albeit Kojic acid was recently removed from the market in Japan due its sensitizing properties.

Licorice extract

Licorice (*Glycyrrhiza glabra, Glycyrrhiza inflate*) extract has been used as a natural remedy for centuries for its anti-inflammatory and anti-irritant properties. Licorice extract derived from the root of *Glycyrrhiza glabra*, glabridin, has dual pigment modulating and anti-inflammatory properties. Active ingredients in licorice extract are the flavenoids, liquirtin and isoliquertin. Licorice extract leads to skin lightening primarily by dispersing melanin.[16] In cultured B16 melanoma cells, glabridin inhibits tyrosinase activity without affecting DNA synthesis rates.[17] Topical application of glabridin has been shown to reduce UVB-induced pigmentation and erythema in the skin of guinea pigs. In vitro anti-inflammatory effects of glabridin relate to inhibition of superoxide production and activity of cyclooxygenase.[17]

For clinical efficacy, glabridin must be applied at a dosage of 1 g/d for at least 4 weeks. Licorice extract is considered a weak lightening agent and must be combined with other agents for optimal clinical results.

Arbutin and deoxyarbutin

Derived from the leaves of the *Vaccinium vitisidaea*, arbutin is a gluconopyranoside that inhibits tyrosinase. It also inhibits melanosome maturation without associated melanocyte toxicity.[18] Arbutin at a concentration of 3% is available in Japan in several over-the-counter preparations. Higher concentrations may provide additional thera-peutic benefit, but paradoxic darkening may occur. Deoxyarbutin is a synthetically modified derivative of arbutin with enhanced pigment lightening properties.[19]

Aloesin

Aloesis is a low-molecular-weight glycoprotein derived from the aloe vera plant. It func-tions through the competitive inhibition of tyrosinase at the dihydroxyphenylalanine (DOPA) oxidation site.[20–22] Therapeutic application of aloesin is limited by its hydro-philic nature and inability to penetrate the skin.

Edelweiss complex

Edelweiss complex is a new approach targeting skin discoloration. It relies on anti-sense oligonucleotides that block targeted gene transcription and modulate melano-genesis. This technology offers unique specificity, biologic stability, and safety in whitening of all skin types. In a clinical study of 30 Asian patients with dyschromia of the hands, the test product applied twice daily for 8 weeks significantly whitened hyperpigmented and normal skin.[23]

Vitamin C

Numerous studies have confirmed the beneficial effects of systemic (oral and intrave-nous [IV] administration[24]) and topically applied ascorbic acid (vitamin C) in the treat-ment of melasma.[5,25,26] In a randomized, split-face clinical trial 16 women were treated with a nightly application of 5% ascorbic acid cream on one side of the face and 4% HQ cream on the opposite side, for 16 weeks.

The HQ and ascorbic acid treated sides had good and excellent results in 93% and 62.5% of patients, respectively. Colorimetric measures showed no statistical differ-ences. Topically applied ascorbic acid was well tolerated with low rates of side effects reported (6.2% vs 68.7% in HQ group).[26]

Vitamin C can also be combined with other treatment modalities such as trichloro-acetic acid (TCA) peel for synergistic effect.[25] One limitation of topically applied ascor-bic acid is its inherent instability (for a detailed discussion see section on Rosacea).

Retinoids

Retinoids are synthetic and natural compounds with structure and activity similar to that of vitamin A. Vitamin A exists as retinol (a vitamin A alcohol), retinal (a vitamin A aldehyde, and retinoic acid (a vitamin A acid). All these forms are inter-convertible. Biologic activity of retinoids relates to their ability to activate RAR $\alpha\beta\gamma$ and RXR $\alpha\beta\gamma$ receptors, and increases from retinol to retinaldehyde to retinoic acid.

A plethora of prescription and over-the-counter retinoids exist. Topical retinoid's ability to depigment is based on its ability to disperse melanosomes, interfere with melanocyte-keratinocyte pigment transfer, and accelerate epidermal turnover and, subsequently, pigment loss.[27,28] In addition, retinoids may inhibit melanogenesis by inhibiting tyrosinase and DOPAchrome conversion factor.[29]

Topical tretinoin (*trans*-retinoic acid) can be effective in the treatment of melasma as monotherapy. In a large-scale, double-blind, placebo-controlled study of 50 white women, topical 0.1% tretinoin caused a marked clinical improvement, 68% and 5% for tretinoin and placebo groups, respectively, at 40 weeks. Clinical improvement was consistent with calorimetric and histologic assessment.[30] Epidermal pigment was reduced by 36% in the tretinoin-treated group.

Overall, the response to tretinoin treatment is less than with HQ and can be slow, with improvement seen after 6 months or longer. Tretinoin as a monotherapy is not an approved treatment of melasma. Nonetheless, a forementioned combination regimen of tretinoin, HQ, and a topical corticosteroid (fluocinolone acetonide) is FDA approved and commercially available as Tri-Luma.[29]

The major adverse effect of retinoids is skin irritation, especially when the more effective, higher concentrations are used. Temporary photosensitivity and paradoxic hyperpigmentation can also occur.

Chemical Peels, Microdermabrasion, Nonablative and Fractional Ablative Light, and Laser Technologies

Chemical peels (superficial peels, including 20%–30% salicylic acid, 30%–40% GA, β-lipohydroxy acid [LHA]), microdermabrasion, and nonablative and fractional ablative technologies[31,32] have been used extensively for the treatment of melasma. Periprocedural use of appropriate cosmeceuticals may enhance postprocedural healing and their continued use may extend the duration of treatment benefits.

A few general principles apply. First, a thorough medical history, including any hypertrophic scarring, viral (herpetic), bacterial (Staphylococcus), and yeast infections, must be obtained. Appropriate antiviral, antibacterial, and antiyeast treatments should be initiated immediately before, and continued for 7 to 10 days following the treatment to prevent infection, as cutaneous infection in the immediate postsurgical period might lead to significant PIH and possible scarring. All medications should be known and oral contraceptives and known photosensitizers should be discontinued if medically possible. Second, medium to high potency topical fluorinated steroids administered 2 to 3 days before treatment and continued for up to 1 to 2 weeks after the treatment might lead to decreased swelling and bleeding. Third, all medications that increase the risk of bleeding (eg, aspirin, nonsteroidal anti-inflammatories, vitamin E, ginkgo) should be stopped unless medically necessary. Fourth, to minimize the risk of scarring and PIH, retinoids or chemical peels should be stopped 3 days (superficial chemical peels) to 2 weeks (nonablative, fractional ablative resurfacing) before the procedure. Systemic isotretinoin should be stopped within 6 (nonablative) to 12 (fractional ablative and ablative) months of the procedure. Fifth, dark-skinned or tanned individuals are at higher risk of postinflammatory dyschromia. The risk of postinflammatory dyschromia after fractional resurfacing may be minimized by pretreatment with HQ.[31]

Postprocedure patients may resume preoperative treatment regimens including depigmenting agents. Following nonablative procedures and fractional ablative procedures, depigmenting agents may be initiated after 1 to 2 weeks or at the first sign of hyperpigmentation. Use of emollients, gentle skin care with toners, and mild cleansers and sun blocks is crucial for optimal healing in the immediate postoperative period.

Laser treatments with Q-switched lasers (neodymium:yttrium-aluminum-garnet [Nd:YAG], frequency-doubled [532 nm] and nonfrequency-doubled [1064 nm]), ruby laser (694 nm), and ablative carbon dioxide and erbium:YAG (2940 nm), seem to show limited usefulness in the treatment of melasma, with high rates of melasma recurrence and a high incidence of PIH.[29]

Recently, fractional resurfacing with a 1550-nm erbium:glass laser (Fraxel SR 750, Reliant Technologies, Inc, Mountain View, CA) has proved to be a promising treatment modality with marked postprocedural clinical, histologic, and ultrastructural improvement.[32–34]

Microdermabrasion

In a large study of 533 patients with melasma, Kunachak and colleagues[35] reported a melasma clearance rate of 97% after microdermabrasion at long-term follow-up.

PIH and postprocedural hyperemia were responsive to 3% to 5% topical HQ or 0.1% triamcinolone.

Chemical Peels

Salicylic acid

Grimes[36] reported moderate to significant improvement of melasma in 4 of 6 patients with skin types V and VI, treated with a series of 20% to 30% salicylic acid (SA) peels (every 2 weeks) plus HQ (administered for 2 weeks before initiation of SA series). The treatment protocol was well tolerated with no reported postinflammatory dyschromia. SA peels without pretreatment with HQ were associated with higher risk of hyperpigmentation (Diane Berson, MD, unpublished observation, personal communication, 2008).

GA

The usefulness of serial GA (an α hydroxyl acid) peels (increasing concentrations 35%, 50%, and 70%) with topical therapy with azaleic acid and adapalene was studied in 28 women with recalcitrant melasma.[37] The combination therapy (GA peels, retinoid, and azaleic acid) group had superior clinical improvement compared with the retinoid plus azaleic acid group. Combined treatment with serial GA peels, azaleic acid cream, and adapalene gel may be an effective and safe therapy for recalcitrant melasma.

Lim and Tham[38] conducted a 26-week, single-blind, split-face study of 10 Asian women treated with GA peels ranging in concentration from 20% to 70%, administered every 3 weeks alone or in combination with topical HQ plus 10% GA. The best clinical improvement was noted in women treated with the combination therapy, although results did not reach statistical significance.

ROSACEA

Introduction

Rosacea is a common, chronic skin disorder that primarily affects the central and convex areas of the face. The nose, cheeks, chin, forehead, and glabella are the most frequently affected sites. The disease has a variety of clinical manifestations ranging from flushing, persistent erythema, telangiectasias, papules, pustules, tissue hyperplasia, and sebaceous gland hyperplasia. Diagnosis of rosacea is based primarily on clinically recognizable morphologic characteristics. An expert committee assembled by the National Rosacea Society on the Classification and Staging of Rosacea defined and classified rosacea in April 2002 into 4 clinical subtypes based primarily on morphologic characteristics. The subtypes include erythematotelangiectatic rosacea, papulopustular rosacea, phymatous rosacea, and ocular rosacea. The pathogenesis of rosacea is complex, with genetic and vascular elements, climatic exposures, matrix degeneration, chemicals and ingested agents, pilosebaceous unit abnormalities, and microbial organisms likely playing a role.[39]

FDA approved rosacea treatment options include systemic and topical antibiotics with antimicrobial and anti-inflammatory properties, azaleic acid, and topical immunomodulators. These medical therapy options are often insufficient, especially for erythematotelangiectatic rosacea motivating patients to search for alternative herbal anti-inflammatories and botanicals. "Anti-red" cosmeceuticals can be combined with prescription medications and in-office procedures.

Anti-inflammatory Botanicals

Licochalcone A (licorice extract)

Licorice extract has marked anti-inflammatory properties. In in vitro studies, licochalcone A isolated from the roots of *Glycyrrhiza inflate* suppresses inflammation via indirect inhibition of the cyclooxygenase (COX) and lipoxygenase pathways. Licochalcone A in vivo decreases UVB-induced erythema, reduces proinflammatory cytokines, and UVB-induced prostaglandin E2 (PGE_2) release by keratinocytes.[17,40] In an 8-week clinical trial of 32 women with mild to moderate rosacea and 30 women with facial erythema, application of 4 test products containing licochalcone A (cleanser, moisturizer with sun protection factor [SPF] 15, spot concealer, and night moisturizing cream) resulted in a significant reduction of erythema at 4 and 8 weeks after initiation of treatment (7% vs 23%, respectively). Licochalcone A-containing cosmeceuticals were well tolerated for everyday use.[40] In another study, topical application of a licochalcone A-containing extract twice daily for 3 days resulted in a significant reduction in UV-induced and shaving-induced erythema.[41]

Azelaic acid
Topical azelaic acid is an FDA approved treatment of rosacea and acne vulgaris and is useful for acne-induced PIH.[42]

Aloe vera
Aloe vera has been widely used in traditional medicine to accelerate healing of wounds and burns. The active ingredients of aloe vera include SA (antimicrobial and anti-inflammatory properties via inhibition of thromboxane and prostaglandin synthesis), magnesium lactate (antipruritic properties via inhibition of histidine decarboxylase), and gel polysaccharides (anti-inflammatory activity by immunomodulation).[43]

The anti-inflammatory properties and clinical efficacy of aloe vera were tested in a double-blind, placebo-controlled trial of 60 patients with mild to moderate psoriasis.[44] Treatment 3 times daily for 5 consecutive days per week for a maximum of 4 weeks with 0.5% aloe vera cream resulted in clearing of psoriatic plaques in 83% of patients compared with only 8% of the placebo group.

Chamomile
Chamomile (Matricaria recutita) has long been used in traditional folk medicine for the treatment of skin irritation and atopic dermatitis. The active components of chamomile include α-bis-abolol, α-bis-abolol oxide A and B, and matricin,[45] all of which are potent inhibitors of COX and lipoxygenase pathways. Chamomile also contains the flavonoids apigenin, luteolin, and quercetin, all potent inhibitors of histamine release.[45] In the skin of healthy volunteers, the anti-inflammatory properties of topical chamomile were comparable with approximately 60% of that produced by hydrocortisone 0.025% cream application.[46]

Feverfew
Feverfew (Tanacetum parthenium) is a nonsteroidal anti-inflammatory agent with marked anti-irritant and antioxidant properties. Anti-inflammatory properties of feverfew include inhibition of proinflammatory cytokine (tumor necrosis factor α [TNFα], interferon-γ [INF-γ], interleukin-2 [IL-2], IL-4) release, decrease in nuclear factor κB (NF-κB) mediated gene transcription, inhibition of neutrophil chemotaxis, and inhibition of adhesion molecule expression.[47] One drawback of topical application of feverfew is a high potential for topical sensitization and irritation. Newly developed purified feverfew extract (Feverfew, PFE) retains the anti-inflammatory properties of feverfew with minimal skin sensitization.

The anti-inflammatory properties of feverfew, as assessed by inhibition of TNFα release, seem to be far superior to other botanicals including teas (green, black, white), echinacea, licorice extract, chamomile, and aloe vera.[47] In a 4-week, controlled, full-face clinical trial, 35 women with mild to moderate facial rosacea were treated with a moisturizing agent containing PFE with an SPF of 15, and a nightly moisturizing cream with PFE, once daily. At 4 weeks, marked improvement in erythema, tactile surface roughness, visual dryness, and overall facial irritation was noted. Application of the feverfew was well tolerated.[4,47] PFE was also shown to reduce UVB-induced erythema in a normal skin. Skin treated for 2 days with 1% PFE and exposed to increasing minimal erythema doses (MEDs; 0.5, 1, 1.5 MED) of UVB showed a marked reduction of erythema at 24 and 48 hours compared with untreated control at all MEDs tested.[48]

Oatmeal

Oatmeal is one of a limited number of natural compounds recognized and regulated by the FDA. Colloidal oatmeal, dehulled oats ground to a fine powder, is recognized by the FDA as a skin protectant that, in addition to providing temporary skin protection, relieves minor pruritus and irritation caused by eczema, rashes, poison ivy, and other contact allergens and insect bites.[49] Colloidal oatmeal has a combination of components and properties well suited for the treatment of inflammatory skin conditions. It cleanses, moisturizes, provides barrier protection, and exhibits anti-inflammatory activity.

The antioxidant constituents of oats are avenanthramides, which are polyphenolic compounds. Isolated avenanthramides reduce proinflammatory cytokines (IL-8) and transcription factors (NF-κB) in cultured human keratinocytes,[50] reduce histamine-induced pruritus in humans, and decrease UVB-induced erythema. In recent months, a topical formulation of proprietary standardized avenanthramide became commercially available as *Avena sativa* kernel.

Pycnogenol

Pycnogenol is a standardized extract from French maritime pine bark (*Pinus pinaster*). The extract's active ingredients include proanthocyanidins, shown to have photoprotective, antimicrobial, antioxidant, anti-inflammatory, and anticarcinogenic effects.[51,52] Its anti-inflammatory properties may include the inhibition of INF-γ and down-regulation of expression of interstitial cell adhesion molecule 1 (ICAM-1) on the surface of keratinocytes. Pycnogenol also converts the vitamin C radical to its active form and raises levels of glutathione and other free-radical scavengers.[3,53] In an animal model, topical application of 0.05% to 0.2% Pycnogenol reduced ultraviolet radiation (UVR)-induced erythema, inflammation, and tumor carcinogenesis in a dose-dependent manner.[52] In a clinical trial of healthy volunteers, 8-week-long oral Pycnogenol supplementation reduced UV-induced erythema.[54]

Lycopene

Lycopene, a carotenoid, exhibits considerable reductive potential and antioxidant activity.[55] When applied topically before UVA exposure, it prevents apoptosis, reduces inflammation, and diminishes expression of enzymes implicated in carcinogenesis.[56] In addition, lycopene has the ability to regenerate vitamin E (α-tocopherol).[55] The clinical usefulness of lycopene still remains to be proved. In a clinical trial of 10 volunteers, 6% topical lycopene cream reduced UV-induced erythema to a greater extent than a topical mixture of vitamin C and vitamin E.[55] In an in vitro study on human fibroblasts exposed to UVA radiation, lycopene offered photoprotection and reduced UVA-induced levels of matrix metalloprotease 1 (MMP-1) only when combined with vitamin E.[56]

Silymarin

Silymarin, a polyphenolic flavonoid from the milk thistle plant, *Silybum marianum*, inhibits lipoprotein oxidation and acts as a free-radical scavenger.[57] In animal models, silymarin showed chemoprotective and anticarcinogenic acitivity.[57,58] It reduced UVB radiation-induced erythema, edema, and keratinocyte apoptosis through the inhibition of inflammatory cytokines and pyrimidine dimers.[59,60] Clinically, silymarin alleviates the symptoms of rosacea. In a double-blinded, placebo-controlled study of 46 patients with rosacea, topical application of silymarin and methylsulfonilmethane for 1 month resulted in statistically significant improvements in erythema, papules, pruritus, and skin hydration.[61]

Quercetin

Found in many fruits and vegetables, the flavonoid quercetin has antioxidant and anti-inflammatory properties. Its anti-inflammatory activity results from inhibition of the enzymatic actions of lipooxygenase and COX-2, and from blocking histamine release. Quercetin also enhances tumor cell apoptosis.[3] In a mouse model, quercetin reduced UVA-induced oxidative stress.[62] In vitro quercetin inhibited growth of melanoma cells.[63]

Allantoin

Allantoin derived from the comfrey root has anti-inflammatory and antioxidant effects. It has been shown to repair cutaneous photodamage and reduce inflammation following UVR exposure.[64]

Chemical Peels

Chemical peels, β-hydroxy acids and α-hydroxy acids (GA) are widely used for the treatment of acne rosacea. Clinical experience has long shown effectiveness of SA in the treatment of acne rosacea. SA targets comedonal and inflammatory lesions and has better sustained efficacy and fewer side effects than GA peels.[65,66]

Lee and colleagues[67] reported improvement in acne in 35 Korean patients treated with 30% SA peels. Grimes[36] reported moderate clearing of inflammatory acne lesions in 8 of 9 dark-skinned patients (diverse ethnicity including subjects of Asian, African, and Hispanic descent) treated with a series of 20% to 30% SA peels with 4% HQ pretreatment. This treatment regimen facilitated resolution of PIH, and a decrease in overall pigmentation of the face.

An SA derivative, lipohydroxyacid (LHA) (commercially available in concentrations up to 10%) has recently been introduced in the United States. With an additional fatty chain, LHA has increased lipophilicity that allows for efficient exfoliation, and increased antibacterial, anti-inflammatory, antifungal, and anticomedogenic properties even at low concentrations.[68] Studies have shown strong keratinolytic properties with good penetration through the epidermis and into the pilosebaceous unit.

In a randomized, controlled clinical trial, Uhoda and colleagues[69] studied LHA peels in acne-prone women and women with comedonal acne. UV light video recordings and computerized image analysis showed significantly decreased numbers and sizes of microcomedones and a reduction in the density of follicular keratotic plugs in the LHA treated group.

Laser Therapy and IPL

Laser therapy with pulsed dye lasers (PDL 585-595 nm), potassium-titanyl-phosphate (KTP), and IPL for acne rosacea has been used extensively for the reduction of telangiectasias, erythema, flushing, and improving skin texture.[70,71] The primary mode of action of laser/ILP therapy is selective photothermolysis of telangiectatic superficial blood vessels.

In a recent small pilot study of 10 rosacea patients treated with either IPL or PDL, 5 patients (3 after IPL and 2 after PDL) had lower levels of cathelicidin, an antimicrobial peptide. Cathelicidins were recently shown to play a central role in the pathogenesis of rosecea.[72] In addition to directly mediating antimicrobial activity, cathelicidins have the potential to trigger the immune host tissue response by promoting leukocyte chemotaxis, angiogenesis, and the expression of components of the extracellular matrix.[73] Patients with rosacea express higher levels of cathelicidins peptides in affected facial areas compared with similar anatomic regions of unaffected controls.

Although the results of the aforementioned trial did not reach statistical significance, the study raised an interesting mechanism for clinical improvement of rosacea symptoms after IPL or laser treatment.[74] Natural anti-inflammatory agents could potentially limit the cathelicidin-medicated inflammatory cascade.

PHOTOAGING (RHYTIDS AND DYSCHROMIA)
Introduction

In the treatment of aging skin, a new generation of cosmeceuticals offers clinical benefits. Ultrapotent antioxidants, stem cell modulators, and antisense DNA technologies are advancing our clinical understanding of the intrinsic and extrinsic aging processes, offering targeted strategies for slowing down or reversing the signs of aging. The aging process has intrinsic and extrinsic bases. These 2 clinically and biologically independent and distinct processes affect skin structure and function.

Intrinsic or innate aging is a naturally occurring process that occurs from slow, but progressive and irreversible, tissue degeneration. Telomere shortening and metabolic oxidative damage with free reactive oxygen species (ROS) generation all play a role in the innate aging process.[75] Based on a unique genetic imprint, intrinsic aging affects everyone at different rates. On a histologic level, intrinsic aging is characterized by decreased collagen synthesis, degeneration of elastic fiber networks, and loss of hydration. Clinically, fine wrinkling of the skin, loss of skin tone, skin laxity, and loss of subcutaneous fat occur.

Of the extrinsic factors, UV and infrared (IR) radiation, environmental pollutants, and physical factors (cold, wind) play a crucial role. UVA radiation is the prime driver of premature aging. Clinically, extrinsic photoaging is characterized by coarse wrinkling and furrowing with an apparent thickening of the skin, elastosis, and a variety of benign, premalignant, and malignant neoplasms.[76] Histologically, photodamaged skin shows a 20% decrease in total collagen and decreased cellular content compared with sun-protected skin.[77] Moreover, pigmentary alterations and telangiectasias contribute to an aged appearance by creating shadows and areas of contrast on the face.

Antioxidants

Antioxidants have long been used in the cosmetic industry for their multifaceted benefits, offering antiaging and anti-inflammatory properties. In addition, antioxidants confer a degree of photoprotection and anticarcinogenesis by quenching free-radical species generated by cellular metabolism and direct exposure to UV radiation. They also block UV-induced inflammatory pathways.

Tea

Tea (black, green, white, oolong) is derived from the leaves and buds of the tea plant (Camellia sinensis). Different varieties of tea result from differential processing, oxidation, and fermentation of the tea leaves and buds.[78] Active ingredients in tea include polyphenolic catechins such as epicatechin, epicatechin-3-gallate (ECG), epigallocatechin (EGC), and epigallocatechin-3-gallate (EGCG).[4]

Green tea offers antioxidant, anti-inflammatory, and anticarcinogenic properties with systemic and topical administration.[79] Early studies on hairless mice fed green tea showed a dose-dependent reduction of UV-induced carcinogenesis.[80,81] Similar anticarcinogenic and chemoprotective effects were shown after topical application of green tea polyphenolic catechins (GTP) in mice. GTP is the active ingredient in green tea and limits UV-induced redness, the number of sunburn cells, collagen, and cellular DNA damage.[81]

In healthy volunteers, topical GTP (EGCG and ECG) inhibited UV-induced erythema and reduced formation of cyclobutane pyrimidine dimers, a marker of DNA damage.[82,83] Green tea has also has been studied for use in cosmetic applications. In a clinical study of 40 women with moderate photoaging, Chin and colleagues found increased elastic tissue content in the skin of women treated with 300 mg of green tea supplements twice daily and topical 10% green tea cream daily. Histologic improvement nonetheless did not correlate with clinical improvement after 8 weeks of treatment, suggesting that (1) histologic improvement (especially mild to moderate) may not translate into short-term clinical improvement, and (2) clinical correlation of all histologic findings is essential.[84]

Vitamin C, vitamin E, and ferulic acid

Cosmeceutical preparations of vitamins C (L-ascorbic acid) and E (D-alpha-tocopherol) play a major role in the treatment of photoaged skin. In vivo, vitamin C blocks UVR-induced erythema. In vitro, vitamin C stimulates fibroblasts, increases rates of neocollagenesis, decreases melanin formation, and exhibits anti-inflammatory activity. The effects of cutaneous vitamin C application were evaluated in a double-blind, half-face trial. A 12-week treatment with vitamin C complex consisting of 10% ascorbic acid (water soluble) and 7% tetrahexyldecyl ascorbate (lipid soluble provitamin C) resulted in significant improvement in photoaging scores and skin wrinkling. Histologic analysis revealed increased collagen content in sites treated with vitamin C complex.[85]

Diet is the sole source of vitamin C in humans. Gastrointestinal absorption is the rate-limiting factor in cutaneous delivery of vitamin C. Therefore, even supraphysiologic doses of vitamin C through oral administration do not increase the cutaneous concentration to optimal levels. Exposure to sunlight and environmental pollutants deplete cutaneous vitamin C. Even minimal UV exposure of 1.6 times the MED decreases the level of vitamin C to 70% of the normal level. Exposure to 10 ppm of ozone in city pollution decreases the level of epidermal vitamin C by 55%.[79]

Vitamin E is the most important lipid soluble, membrane-bound antioxidant in plasma, cellular membranes, and tissues. Similar to vitamin C, vitamin E is supplied solely through diet. In animal studies, vitamin E, decreases the rate of UVR-induced tumor formation. In clinical studies, topically applied vitamin E decreased the appearance of wrinkles, solar lentigines, and overall photoaging.

In tissues, vitamins C and E act synergistically to provide antioxidant protection. When used in combination, topical L-ascorbic acid (15%) and D-α-tocopherol (1%) resulted in a fourfold greater protection against UV-induced erythema, compared with a twofold increase with either agent alone.

The inherent instability of active vitamin C (L-ascorbic acid), however, remains the major therapeutic challenge. When exposed to air, L-ascorbic acid converts to inactive brown dihydroascorbic acid. To overcome the problem of instability, vitamin C and vitamin E preparations have been stabilized with ferulic acid. Ferulic acid is a potent antioxidant present in the cell walls of grains, fruits, and vegetables. The acid itself absorbs UV radiation, acting as a sunscreen. When mixed with vitamins E and C, it stabilizes the formulation and doubles synergistic photoprotection from fourfold (combined vitamins C and E) to eightfold (vitamin C, vitamin E, ferulic acid; C E ferulic).[80] Clinical studies show that topical C E ferulic acid provides substantial protection for human skin against solar simulator-induced oxidative skin damage, including erythema, sunburn cell formation, and cancer related DNA mutations.[86]

Yquem

Yquem extract is a novel, highly potent antioxidant. In in vitro studies it has been shown to cause highly significant reduction of oxidative stress. The antioxidant power of yquem extract at low concentrations (1.5 μg/mL) is highly superior to that of vitamin C (at 50 μM) and that of vitamin E (at 25μM). In a clinical study of 10 subjects, the extract was applied for 1 day to facial skin, and the rates of free-radical production were measured 18 hours after the last application and compared with an untreated zone. Treatment with yquem extract decreased the rate of free-radical production by 22% compared with untreated control. By comparison, grape polyphenols and idebendone formulations decreased free-radical production by only 2.3% and 4.1%, respectively.[9]

Coffeeberry

Polyphenols including chlorogenic acid, quinic acid, ferulic acid, and condensed proanthocyanidins are the active ingredients in coffeeberry, the fruit of the coffee plant *Coffea arabica*.[87] The antioxidant properties of polyphenols are related to their ability to quench free radicals. In in vitro testing with the oxygen radical absorbance capacity (ORAC) assay, coffeeberry was superior to other commonly used antioxidants, such as green tea extract, pomegranate extract, vitamin C, and vitamin E.[81,88] The clinical relevance of in vitro ORAC testing is controversial, especially because the ORAC scale was originally developed to determine the antioxidant potential of ingested, rather than topically applied, antioxidants.[89]

In a 6-week double-blind clinical trial, 30 patients with significant actinic damage used a skin regimen of 0.1% to 1% coffeeberry in skin cleansers and facial creams (commercially available as the RevaléSkin line, Stiefel). Compared with pretreatment, all patients saw statistically significant improvements in fine lines, wrinkles, pigmentation, and overall skin appearance[88]

Idebenone

This is a low-molecular-weight synthetic analog of coenzyme Q10. Because of its lower molecular weight, idebenone can penetrate the skin more efficiently than coenzyme Q10. In a clinical study of 50 subjects with moderate photoaging, an application of 0.5% to 1% idebenone lotion twice daily for 6 weeks reduced fine lines and wrinkles by 26% and 27%, respectively. Both groups saw a 37% improvement in skin hydration and a 30% to 33% improvement in global photoaging.[90]

Vine shoot

A new generation of ultrapotent antioxidants include *Vitis vinifera* shoot, a polyphenol-rich antioxidant and ectoine/hydroine, a natural blend of compounds found in halophilic microorganisms growing in extreme temperature and salinity. In a clinical study, 56 subjects were treated with a combination of *Vitis vinifera* shoot extract (0.045%) and ectoine/hydroine (1%). The combination was applied for a 4-week period twice daily; 90% of patients experienced a 25% overall improvement (firmness, radiant glow, evenness, smoothness, hydration, texture, softness) as assessed by an independent investigator. In in vitro assays, the antioxidant capacity of *Vitis vinifera* shoot appeared to be significantly more powerful than that of vitamin C or E.[91]

Soy

Isoflavones, including genistein and diadzein, are the main active ingredients and chemoprotective agents derived from soy. Other biologically active ingredients include essential fatty acids and amino acids, phytosterols, and small protein serine protease inhibitors such as Bowman-Birk inhibitor (BBI) and soy trypsin inhibitor (STI). By inhibiting protease-activated receptor 2 (PAR-2), STI inhibits melanosome transfer to keratinocytes.[92] Clinically, soy provides gentle anti-inflammatory, photoprotective, and skin lightening properties. Daily, or twice daily, application of a topical soy formulation over a 12-week period resulted in improved overall skin tone and texture, hyperpigmentation, skin blotchiness, and dullness (Diane Berson, MD, personal communication, 2009). In a clinical study of 6 adult patients, genistein showed a dose-dependent inhibition of UBV-induced erythema.[93]

Sunscreens

Broad-spectrum UVA and UVB sunscreens are the cornerstone of photoaging therapy. UVR causes several acute effects in the skin, including photosynthesis of vitamin D, immediate pigment darkening, delayed tanning, sunburn, epidermal thickening, and numerous immunologic effects, from altered antigen presentation to release of immunosuppressive factors.

UVA and UVB radiation contribute to the disruption of the extracellular matrix, a hallmark of photoaging. The presence of dermal changes in the deep reticular dermis, however, suggests that UVA radiation plays a key role, because only a small percentage of UVB penetrates into the superficial papillary dermis.[94,95] The mechanism of UVR mediated dermal damage includes:

1. Decreased collagen I and III synthesis
2. Increased collagen degradation by transforming growth factor-β (TGF-β) and activator protein A
3. Infiltration of inflammatory cells, predominately neutrophils, into the dermis
4. Release of ROS from neutrophils.

Benzophenones (dioxybenzone, oxybenzone, sulisobenzone) provide protection in the UVB and UVA II range (320–340 nm). Currently, only oxybenzone is approved for use in the United States.

Avobenzone (Parson 1789), a dibenzoylmethane, absorbs in the UVA I (340–400 nm) range. However, its use is limited by its relative instability. Estimates suggest that all avobenzone is inactivated after 5 hours of sun exposure, equivalent to 50 J of solar energy. Stability of the avobenzone is markedly increased by combining with oxybenzone and 2,6-diethylhexylnaphthalate in commercially available Helioplex (Neutrogena). Another agent offering long-lasting short-wave UVA protection and photostabilization of avobenzone is ecamsule, commercially available as Mexoryl (L'Oreal, France).

Retinoids

The biologic properties of retinoids include free-radical scavenging and antioxidant activity, increasing fibroblast proliferation, modulation of cellular proliferation and differentiation, increased collagen and hyaluronate synthesis, and decreased matrix metalloproteinase mediated extracellular matrix degradation. Retinoids are therefore ideal for the treatment of photoaging.[96] Numerous studies have confirmed the clinical efficacy of various retinoids.[27,96–101] Histologic responses to chronic topical retinoid application include hyperproliferation, leading to a dose-dependent expansion of the numbers of cell layers of stratum spinosum and stratum granulosum, and elongation of the basal layer keratinocytes.

Chemical Peels

The efficacy of chemical peels for the treatment of photodamage has been widely reported.[102,103] Histologically, different chemical peels, GA, SA and LHA, alter the epidermis toward a non–sun-damaged pattern with keratinocytes showing a return of polarity, and more regular distribution of melanocytes and melanin granules.

In a randomized, right/left split-face controlled clinical trial of 43 women aged 35 to 60 years with fine lines, wrinkles, and dyschromia, application of 4 LHA (5%–10%) treatments was equivalent to 6 treatment sessions with GA (20%–50%). Both chemical peels were well tolerated and showed a significant reduction of all study parameters (fine lines, wrinkles, and hyperpigmentation) (LaRoche Posay, 2008, clinical data on file).

Laser Skin Resurfacing

The carbon dioxide and Er:YAG lasers remain gold standard for rejuvenation of photoaged skin. However, their use is associated with a risk of side effects and a prolonged postoperative recovery period. Newer rejuvenating laser systems offer the benefit of stimulation of collagen production and remodeling with little or no healing time and decreased patient discomfort.

Nonablative laser systems currently available include:

1. Mid-IR lasers targeting the dermis (Nd:YAG [1320 nm], diode [1450 μm])
2. Visible lasers, such as the PDL (585-595 nm) the pulsed KTP (532 nm) and Nd:YAG (1064 nm)
3. IPL
4. A combination of electrical (radiofrequency) and optical devices.

Fractional resurfacing offers partial benefits of the ablative laser with faster recovery and fewer side effects. In addition to the original Fraxel SR (1550 nm erbium, Reliant Technologies), the Fraxel SR1500, Fraxel AFR (both Reliant Technologies), Lux 1540 Fractional (1540 nm, Palomar Medical Technologies, Burlington, MA, USA), and Affirm (1320 nm plus 1440 nm, Cynosure Inc, Westford, MA, USA) have been developed.[104]

COLLAGEN REPAIR
Introduction

The use of signaling peptides, growth factors (GF) and cytokines in collagen repair and clinical rejuvenation has emerged as an exciting new antiaging treatment option. Advances in basic research into wound healing, with the identification of key wound healing mediators, prompted translational clinical research on repair and remodeling of dermal infrastructure. The GFs implicated in wound healing are listed in **Table 1**.

GFs

Cell rejuvenation serum (CRS, Topix Pharmaceuticals, NY, USA) relies on liposomal technology for dermal delivery of TGF-β1, L-ascorbic acid, and black cohosh (*Cimicifuga racemosa*). In a split-face clinical study of 12 patients with moderate facial photoaging, patients applied CRS cream with TGF-β1 to one side of the face and CRS cream without TGF-β1 to the opposite side. The results showed a statistically

Table 1 GF and cytokine signals involved in wound healing	
GF	**Cell Target and Effect**
Heparin-binding epidermal growth factor-like growth factor (HB-EGF)	Keratinocyte and fibroblast mitogen
Fibroblastic growth factor (FGF) 1, 2, 4	Angiogenic, fibroblast mitogen
Platelet-derived growth factor (PDGF)	Chemotaxis of macrophages and fibroblasts; macrophage activation; fibroblasts mitogen, matrix production
Insulin-like growth factor 1 (IGF-1)	Endothelial cells and fibroblast mitogen
TGF-β1 and β2	Keratinocyte migration; chemotaxis for macrophages and fibroblast
TGF-β3	Antiscarring
IL-1α and -β	Early activators of GF expression in macrophages, keratinocytes and fibroblasts
TNF α	Mechanism of action similar to IL-1α and -β

Data from Mehta RC, Fitzpatrick RE. Endogenous growth factors as cosmeceuticals. Dermatol Ther 2007;20(5):350–9.

significant improvement of facial rhytids with the CRS cream containing TGF-β1 compared with the L-ascorbic acid and black cohosh only CRS preparation.[105]

NouriCel-MD, a proprietary mix of GFs, cytokines, and soluble proteins secreted by cultured neonatal human dermal fibroblasts during production of extracellular matrix in an oil-free gel, is currently available as TNS Recovery Complex (SkinMedica Inc, Carlsbad, CA, USA). In a clinical study, 14 patients with marked photodamage applied TNS Recovery Complex twice daily to facial skin for 60 days. The results showed a 15% to 35% decrease in fine lines and wrinkles as assessed by optical profilometry assay. In addition, thickening of the Grenz zone, new collagen formation (average 36%) and epidermal thickening (average 30%) were noted.[106]

The main ingredients in Bio-Restorative Skin Cream (Neocutis, Inc, San Francisco, CA, USA) are processed skin-cell proteins, a proprietary blend of GFs, and cytokines extracted from cultured first trimester fetal human dermal fibroblasts. Compared with adult fibroblasts, fetal fibroblasts express only transient and low amounts of TGF-β1, which may contribute to virtually scarless healing in the first trimester of pregnancy.[107] Clinical benefits of Bio-Restorative Skin Cream were studied in 18 patients with moderate to severe photodamage. Twice daily application of Bio-Restorative Skin Cream for 60 days resulted in a 17% and 13% decrease in periorbital and perioral rhytids. Improvements in skin texture were also noted.[108]

Peptides

Cosmeceutical peptides, short-chain sequences of amino acids, are a rapidly expanding category of cosmeceuticals. Biologic effects of peptides may relate to their ability to enhance collagen production, relax dynamic skin wrinkling, and improve skin hydration and barrier function. The three main classes of peptides are signal peptides, neuropeptides, and carrier peptides.

Signal peptides

Signal peptides increase fibroblast production of collagen or decrease collagenase breakdown of existing collagen. Examples of signal peptides include valine-glycine-alanine-proline-glycine   peptide,[109,110]   lysine-threonine-threonine-lysine-serine peptide (KTTKS),[111] tyrosine-tyrosine-arginine-alanine-aspartame-aspartame-alanine peptide, and glycyl-L-histadyl-L-lysine (GHK) peptide.

Application of elastin-derived valine-glycine-alanine-proline-glycine peptide has been shown to significantly stimulate human dermal skin fibroblast production and down-regulate elastin expression. Palmitate-bound valine-glycine-alanine-proline-glycine peptide is commercially available in a number of cosmetic preparations under the trade name of palmitoyl oligopeptide.[2]

Palmitate-bound KTTKS peptide (pal-KTTKS, palmitoyl pentapeptide-3, trade name Matrixyl, Sederma, France) is a fragment of type I procollagen. Of the many collagen breakdown products, pentapeptide KTTKS was shown to have the highest fibroblast stimulation properties in in vitro subconfluent monolayer cultures. Exposure of fibroblasts to collagen degradation products is hypothesized to induce cellular collagen repair with enhanced collagen synthesis and down-regulation of matrix collagenases. Pentapeptide was shown to stimulate new collagen synthesis and increase production of extracellular matrix proteins such as type I and II collagen and fibronectin.[112] Matrixyl contains 800 parts per million of pal-KTTKS, and currently available cosmetic preparations contain 1 to 4 parts per million of pal-KTTKS.[6] In a 12-week double-blind, placebo-controlled, split-face study of 93 Caucasian women, pal-KTTKS provided significant improvement of wrinkles and fine lines compared with the placebo group by qualitative technical and expert grader image analysis.[113]

Neuropeptides

Also known as neurotransmitter-affecting peptides, neuropeptides mimic the effects of botulinum neurotoxin. Clinically, neuropeptides decrease facial muscle contraction, reducing lines and wrinkles by raising the threshold for minimal muscle activity. Over time, they are postulated to also reduce subconscious muscle movement. The properties of several neuropeptides are discussed below. For a comprehensive review see Lupo and colleagues.[2]

Neuropeptides are designed to block individual components of the neuromuscular junction (NMJ). Most neuropeptides act on the soluble N-ethylmaleimide-sensitive factor attachment protein receptors (SNARE) complex, a component of the NMJ. Whether topically applied neuropeptides can truly penetrate to the level of the NMJ remains to be tested.

Acetyl-hexapeptide-3 (AC-gly glu-met-gln-arg-arg-NH_2) is a synthetic peptide patterned after the N-terminus of SNAP-25, an inhibitor of SNARE complex formation and catecholamine release. This peptide is currently marketed as Argireline (McEit International Trade Co, Ltd).[114] In one open-label trial, 10 female patients applied a 5% acetyl-hexapeptide-3 cream twice daily. Subjects experienced a 27% improvement in periorbital rhytids after 30 days as measured by silica replica analysis.[114]

Pentapetide-3 (amino acid sequence not published), currently marketed as Vialox (Cellular Skin, Rx) has a mechanism of action similar to that of tubocurarine, the main ingredient of curare. Its mechanism of action is competitive inhibition of acetylcholine postsynaptic membrane receptor. Acetylcholine receptor blockage in turn prevents muscle contraction.[2]

Carrier peptides

Carrier peptides stabilize and deliver trace elements necessary for wound healing, enzymatic processes, and collagen regeneration into the skin. The most commonly encountered carrier peptides stabilize and deliver copper, an elemental metal for proper wound healing, enzymatic processes (collagen and elastin synthesis, cytochrome c oxidase, down-regulation of MMPs and inhibition of collagenase), and cutaneous aniogenesis.[2] The copper peptide technology is currently adapted for antiaging and general skin care in several skin care preparations. The tripeptide complex, GHK spontaneously complexes with copper and facilities its cellular uptake.[115] In vitro GHK-copper complex increases levels of tissue inhibitors of MMPs, stimulates collagen I and glycosoaminoglycans synthesis, and enzymatic actions of cytochrome c oxidase and tyrosinase.[116] Clinically, GHK-copper application led to an improvement in the appearance of fine lines/wrinkles and an increase in skin density and skin thickeness.[2]

Nonablative, Fractional and Ablative Laser Resurfacing

Cosmeceuticals directed at collagen repair may prove to be of pivotal importance when combined with nonablative, fractional, and ablative laser resurfacing. Laser resurfacing rejuvenates skin by producing controlled zones of dermal or epidermal wounding (epidermal damage is not seen with nonablative technologies). Subsequent inflammation and cytokine mediated superficial dermal healing and remodeling leads to clinical improvement. Application of GFs and collagen repair peptides might further accelerate or improve the wound healing process. Fractional and ablative, compared with nonablative, resurfacing provides an additional benefit of altering the barrier properties of the epidermis and may allow for enhanced penetration of GF and peptides in the immediate postoperative period. That, in theory, may offer deeper penetration and pandermal rejuvenation. Preprocedural treatment with GF and peptides may prime the skin, allowing for a more robust rejuvenating response to laser resurfacing.

REFERENCES

1. Kligman A. The future of cosmeceuticals: an interview with Albert Kligman, MD, PhD. Interview by Zoe Diana Draelos. Dermatol Surg 2005;31(7 Pt 2):890–1.
2. Lupo MP, Cole AL. Cosmeceutical peptides. Dermatol Ther 2007;20(5):343–9.
3. Choi CM, Berson DS. Cosmeceuticals. Semin Cutan Med Surg 2006;25(3): 163–8.
4. Berson DS. Natural antioxidants. J Drugs Dermatol 2008;7(7 Suppl):s7–12.
5. Draelos ZD. Skin lightening preparations and the hydroquinone controversy. Dermatol Ther 2007;20(5):308–13.
6. Draelos ZD. The cosmeceutical realm. Clin Dermatol 2008;26(6):627–32.
7. Draelos ZD. Topical agents used in association with cosmetic surgery. Semin Cutan Med Surg 1999;18(2):112–8.
8. Lawrence N, Bligard CA, Reed R, et al. Exogenous ochronosis in the United States. J Am Acad Dermatol 1988;18(5 Pt 2):1207–11.
9. Westerhof W, Kooyers TJ. Hydroquinone and its analogues in dermatology – a potential health risk. J Cosmet Dermatol 2005;4(2):55–9.
10. Fitton A, Goa KL. Azelaic acid. A review of its pharmacological properties and therapeutic efficacy in acne and hyperpigmentary skin disorders. Drugs 1991; 41(5):780–98.
11. Balina LM, Graupe K. The treatment of melasma. 20% azelaic acid versus 4% hydroquinone cream. Int J Dermatol 1991;30(12):893–5.
12. Bissett D. Topical niacinamide and barrier enhancement. Cutis 2002;70(6 Suppl):8–12.
13. Bissett DL, Oblong JE, Berge CA. Niacinamide: A B vitamin that improves aging facial skin appearance. Dermatol Surg 2005;31(7 Pt 2):860–5.

14. Greatens A, Hakozaki T, Koshoffer A, et al. Effective inhibition of melanosome transfer to keratinocytes by lectins and niacinamide is reversible. Exp Dermatol 2005;14(7):498–508.
15. Bissett DL, Robinson LR, Raleigh PS, et al. Reduction in the appearance of facial hyperpigmentation by topical N-acetyl glucosamine. J Cosmet Dermatol 2007;6(1):20–6.
16. Amer M, Metwalli M. Topical liquiritin improves melasma. Int J Dermatol 2000; 39(4):299–301.
17. Yokota T, Nishio H, Kubota Y, et al. The inhibitory effect of glabridin from licorice extracts on melanogenesis and inflammation. Pigment Cell Res 1998;11(6): 355–61.
18. Hori I, Nihei K, Kubo I. Structural criteria for depigmenting mechanism of arbutin. Phytother Res 2004;18(6):475–9.
19. Hamed SH, Sriwiriyanont P, deLong MA, et al. Comparative efficacy and safety of deoxyarbutin, a new tyrosinase-inhibiting agent. J Cosmet Sci 2006;57(4): 291–308.
20. Choi S, Lee SK, Kim JE, et al. Aloesin inhibits hyperpigmentation induced by UV radiation. Clin Exp Dermatol 2002;27(6):513–5.
21. Jones K, Hughes J, Hong M, et al. Modulation of melanogenesis by aloesin: a competitive inhibitor of tyrosinase. Pigment Cell Res 2002;15(5):335–40.
22. Wang Z, Li X, Yang Z, et al. Effects of aloesin on melanogenesis in pigmented skin equivalents. Int J Cosmet Sci 2008;30(2):121–30.
23. Lazou K, Sadick NS, Kurfurst R, et al. The use of antisense strategy to modulate human melanogenesis. J Drugs Dermatol 2007;6(Suppl 6):s2–7.
24. Lee GS. Intravenous vitamin C in the treatment of post-laser hyperpigmentation for melasma: a short report. J Cosmet Laser Ther 2008;10(4):234–6.
25. Soliman MM, Ramadan SA, Bassiouny DA, et al. Combined trichloroacetic acid peel and topical ascorbic acid versus trichloroacetic acid peel alone in the treatment of melasma: a comparative study. J Cosmet Dermatol 2007;6(2):89–94.
26. Espinal-Perez LE, Moncada B, Castanedo-Cazares JP. A double-blind randomized trial of 5% ascorbic acid vs. 4% hydroquinone in melasma. Int J Dermatol 2004;43(8):604–7.
27. Kaidbey KH, Kligman AM, Yoshida H. Effects of intensive application of retinoic acid on human skin. Br J Dermatol 1975;92(6):693–701.
28. Kligman AM, Willis I. A new formula for depigmenting human skin. Arch Dermatol 1975;111(1):40–8.
29. Gupta AK, Gover MD, Nouri K, et al. The treatment of melasma: a review of clinical trials. J Am Acad Dermatol 2006;55(6):1048–65.
30. Griffiths CE, Finkel LJ, Ditre CM, et al. Topical tretinoin (retinoic acid) improves melasma. A vehicle-controlled, clinical trial. Br J Dermatol 1993;129(4):415–21.
31. Rahman Z, Alam M, Dover JS. Fractional laser treatment for pigmentation and texture improvement. Skin Therapy Lett 2006;11(9):7–11.
32. Goldberg DJ, Berlin AL, Phelps R. Histologic and ultrastructural analysis of melasma after fractional resurfacing. Lasers Surg Med 2008;40(2):134–8.
33. Tannous ZS, Astner S. Utilizing fractional resurfacing in the treatment of therapy-resistant melasma. J Cosmet Laser Ther 2005;7(1):39–43.
34. Rokhsar CK, Fitzpatrick RE. The treatment of melasma with fractional photothermolysis: a pilot study. Dermatol Surg 2005;31(12):1645–50.
35. Kunachak S, Leelaudomlipi P, Wongwaisayawan S. Dermabrasion: a curative treatment for melasma. Aesthetic Plast Surg 2001;25(2):114–7.

36. Grimes PE. The safety and efficacy of salicylic acid chemical peels in darker racial-ethnic groups. Dermatol Surg 1999;25(1):18–22.
37. Erbil H, Sezer E, Tastan B, et al. Efficacy and safety of serial glycolic acid peels and a topical regimen in the treatment of recalcitrant melasma. J Dermatol 2007; 34(1):25–30.
38. Lim JT, Tham SN. Glycolic acid peels in the treatment of melasma among Asian women. Dermatol Surg 1997;23(3):177–9.
39. Reszko AE, Granstein. Pathogenesis of rosacea. J Cosmet Dermatol 2008; 21(4):224–32.
40. Weber TM, Ceilley RI, Buerger A, et al. Skin tolerance, efficacy, and quality of life of patients with red facial skin using a skin care regimen containing Licochalcone A. J Cosmet Dermatol 2006;5(3):227–32.
41. Kolbe L, Immeyer J, Batzer J, et al. Anti-inflammatory efficacy of Licochalcone A: correlation of clinical potency and in vitro effects. Arch Dermatol Res 2006; 298(1):23–30.
42. Del Rosso JQ. The use of topical azelaic acid for common skin disorders other than inflammatory rosacea. Cutis 2006;77(Suppl 2):22–4.
43. Bedi MK, Shenefelt PD. Herbal therapy in dermatology. Arch Dermatol 2002; 138(2):232–42.
44. Syed TA, Ahmad SA, Holt AH, et al. Management of psoriasis with aloe vera extract in a hydrophilic cream: a placebo-controlled, double-blind study. Trop Med Int Health 1996;1(4):505–9.
45. Brown DJ, Dattner AM. Phytotherapeutic approaches to common dermatologic conditions. Arch Dermatol 1998;134(11):1401–4.
46. Albring M, Albrecht H, Alcorn G, et al. The measuring of the antiinflammatory effect of a compound on the skin of volunteers. Methods Find Exp Clin Pharmacol 1983;5(8):575–7.
47. Wu J. Anti-inflammatory ingredients. J Drugs Dermatol 2008;7(Suppl 7):s13–6.
48. Martin K, Sur R, Liebel F, et al. Parthenolide-depleted feverfew (Tanacetum parthenium) protects skin from UV irradiation and external aggression. Arch Dermatol Res 2008;300(2):69–80.
49. FDA, Department of Health and Human Services [HHS]. Skin protectant drug products for over-the-counter human use; final monograph. Final rule. Fed Regist 2003;68(33):362–81.
50. Kurtz ES, Wallo W. Colloidal oatmeal: history, chemistry and clinical properties. J Drugs Dermatol 2007;6(2):167–70.
51. Torras MA, Faura CA, Schonlau F, et al. Antimicrobial activity of Pycnogenol. Phytother Res 2005;19(7):647–8.
52. Sime S, Reeve VE. Protection from inflammation, immunosuppression and carcinogenesis induced by UV radiation in mice by topical Pycnogenol. Photochem Photobiol 2004;79(2):193–8.
53. Rohdewald P. A review of the French maritime pine bark extract (Pycnogenol), a herbal medication with a diverse clinical pharmacology. Int J Clin Pharmacol Ther 2002;40(4):158–68.
54. Saliou C, Rimbach G, Moini H, et al. Solar ultraviolet-induced erythema in human skin and nuclear factor-kappa-B-dependent gene expression in keratinocytes are modulated by a French maritime pine bark extract. Free Radic Biol Med 2001;30(2):154–60.
55. Andreassi M, Stanghellini E, Ettorre A, et al. Antioxidant activity of topically applied lycopene. J Eur Acad Dermatol Venereol 2004;18(1):52–5.

56. Offord EA, Gautier JC, Avanti O, et al. Photoprotective potential of lycopene, beta-carotene, vitamin E, vitamin C and carnosic acid in UVA-irradiated human skin fibroblasts. Free Radic Biol Med 2002;32(12):1293–303.

57. Pinnell SR. Cutaneous photodamage, oxidative stress, and topical antioxidant protection. J Am Acad Dermatol 2003;48(1):1–19.

58. Singh RP, Agarwal R. Flavonoid antioxidant silymarin and skin cancer. Antioxid Redox Signal 2002;4(4):655–63.

59. Katiyar SK, Roy AM, Baliga MS. Silymarin induces apoptosis primarily through a p53-dependent pathway involving Bcl-2/Bax, cytochrome c release, and caspase activation. Mol Cancer Ther 2005;4(2):207–16.

60. Katiyar SK. Silymarin and skin cancer prevention: anti-inflammatory, antioxidant and immunomodulatory effects [review]. Int J Oncol 2005;26(1):169–76.

61. Berardesca E, Cameli N, Cavallotti C, et al. Combined effects of silymarin and methylsulfonylmethane in the management of rosacea: clinical and instrumental evaluation. J Cosmet Dermatol 2008;7(1):8–14.

62. Erden IM, Kahraman A, Koken T. Beneficial effects of quercetin on oxidative stress induced by ultraviolet A. Clin Exp Dermatol 2001;26(6):536–9.

63. Piantelli M, Maggiano N, Ricci R, et al. Tamoxifen and quercetin interact with type II estrogen binding sites and inhibit the growth of human melanoma cells. J Invest Dermatol 1995;105(2):248–53.

64. Thornfeldt C. Cosmeceuticals containing herbs: fact, fiction, and future. Dermatol Surg 2005;31(7 Pt 2):873–80.

65. Taub AF. Procedural treatments for acne vulgaris. Dermatol Surg 2007;33(9):1005–26.

66. Kessler E, Flanagan K, Chia C, et al. Comparison of alpha- and beta-hydroxy acid chemical peels in the treatment of mild to moderately severe facial acne vulgaris. Dermatol Surg 2008;34(1):45–50.

67. Lee HS, Kim IH. Salicylic acid peels for the treatment of acne vulgaris in Asian patients. Dermatol Surg 2003;29(12):1196–9.

68. Corcuff P, Fiat F, Minondo AM, et al. A comparative ultrastructural study of hydroxyacids induced desquamation. Eur J Dermatol 2002;12(4). XXXIX–XLIII.

69. Uhoda E, Pierard-Franchimont C, Pierard GE. Comedolysis by a lipohydroxyacid formulation in acne-prone subjects. Eur J Dermatol 2003;13(1):65–8.

70. Lowe NJ, Behr KL, Fitzpatrick R, et al. Flash lamp pumped dye laser for rosacea-associated telangiectasia and erythema. J Dermatol Surg Oncol 1991;17(6):522–5.

71. Butterwick KJ, Butterwick LS, Han A. Laser and light therapies for acne rosacea. J Drugs Dermatol 2006;5(1):35–9.

72. Yamasaki K, Di NA, Bardan A, et al. Increased serine protease activity and cathelicidin promotes skin inflammation in rosacea. Nat Med 2007;13(8):975–80.

73. Barak O, Treat JR, James WD. Antimicrobial peptides: effectors of innate immunity in the skin. Adv Dermatol 2005;21:357–74.

74. Harvey J. Rosacea: molecular insights. Skin Aging 2007;14.

75. Kosmadaki MG, Gilchrest BA. The role of telomeres in skin aging/photoaging. Micron 2004;35(3):155–9.

76. Gilchrest BA. Skin aging and photoaging: an overview. J Am Acad Dermatol 1989;21(3 Pt 2):610–3.

77. Schwartz E, Cruickshank FA, Christensen CC, et al. Collagen alterations in chronically sun-damaged human skin. Photochem Photobiol 1993;58(6):841–4.

78. Camouse MM, Hanneman KK, Conrad EP, et al. Protective effects of tea polyphenols and caffeine. Expert Rev Anticancer Ther 2005;5(6):1061–8.

79. Katiyar SK, Elmets CA, Agarwal R, et al. Protection against ultraviolet-B radiation-induced local and systemic suppression of contact hypersensitivity and edema responses in C3H/HeN mice by green tea polyphenols. Photochem Photobiol 1995;62(5):855–61.

80. Wang ZY, Agarwal R, Bickers DR, et al. Protection against ultraviolet B radiation-induced photocarcinogenesis in hairless mice by green tea polyphenols. Carcinogenesis 1991;12(8):1527–30.

81. Vayalil PK, Mittal A, Hara Y, et al. Green tea polyphenols prevent ultraviolet light-induced oxidative damage and matrix metalloproteinases expression in mouse skin. J Invest Dermatol 2004;122(6):1480–7.

82. Katiyar SK, Afaq F, Perez A, et al. Green tea polyphenol (−)-epigallocatechin-3-gallate treatment of human skin inhibits ultraviolet radiation-induced oxidative stress. Carcinogenesis 2001;22(2):287–94.

83. Elmets CA, Singh D, Tubesing K, et al. Cutaneous photoprotection from ultraviolet injury by green tea polyphenols. J Am Acad Dermatol 2001;44(3):425–32.

84. Chiu AE, Chan JL, Kern DG, et al. Double-blinded, placebo-controlled trial of green tea extracts in the clinical and histologic appearance of photoaging skin. Dermatol Surg 2005;31(7 Pt 2):855–60.

85. Fitzpatrick RE, Rostan EF. Double-blind, half-face study comparing topical vitamin C and vehicle for rejuvenation of photodamage. Dermatol Surg 2002; 28(3):231–6.

86. Lin FH, Lin JY, Gupta RD, et al. Ferulic acid stabilizes a solution of vitamins C and E and doubles its photoprotection of skin. J Invest Dermatol 2005;125(4): 826–32.

87. Baumann LS. Less-known botanical cosmeceuticals. Dermatol Ther 2007;20(5): 330–42.

88. Farris P. Idebenone, green tea, and coffeeberry extract: new and innovative antioxidants. Dermatol Ther 2007;20(5):322–9.

89. Ditre C, Wu J, Baumann LS, et al. Innovations in natural antioxidants and their role in dermatology. Cutis 2008;82(6 Suppl):2–16.

90. McDaniel D, Neudecker B, Dinardo J, et al. Clinical efficacy assessment in photodamaged skin of 0.5% and 1.0% idebenone. J Cosmet Dermatol 2005;4(3): 167–73.

91. Cornacchione S, Sadick NS, Neveu M, et al. In vivo skin antioxidant effect of a new combination based on a specific *Vitis vinifera* shoot extract and a biotechnological extract. J Drugs Dermatol 2007;6(Suppl 6):s8–13.

92. Seiberg M, Paine C, Sharlow E, et al. The protease-activated receptor 2 regulates pigmentation via keratinocyte-melanocyte interactions. Exp Cell Res 2000;254(1):25–32.

93. Wei H, Saladi R, Lu Y, et al. Isoflavone genistein: photoprotection and clinical implications in dermatology. J Nutr 2003;133(11 Suppl 1):3811S–9S.

94. Lim HH, Buttery JE. Determination of ethanol in serum by an enzymatic PMS-INT colorimetric method. Clin Chim Acta 1977;75(1):9–12.

95. Talwar HS, Griffiths CE, Fisher GJ, et al. Reduced type I and type III procollagens in photodamaged adult human skin. J Invest Dermatol 1995;105(2): 285–90.

96. Sorg O, Kuenzli S, Kaya G, et al. Proposed mechanisms of action for retinoid derivatives in the treatment of skin aging. J Cosmet Dermatol 2005;4(4):237–44.

97. Stefanaki C, Stratigos A, Katsambas A. Topical retinoids in the treatment of photoaging. J Cosmet Dermatol 2005;4(2):130–4.
98. Singh M, Griffiths CE. The use of retinoids in the treatment of photoaging. Dermatol Ther 2006;19(5):297–305.
99. Serri R, Iorizzo M. Cosmeceuticals: focus on topical retinoids in photoaging. Clin Dermatol 2008;26(6):633–5.
100. Mukherjee S, Date A, Patravale V, et al. Retinoids in the treatment of skin aging: an overview of clinical efficacy and safety. Clin Interv Aging 2006;1(4):327–48.
101. Helfrich YR, Sachs DL, Voorhees JJ. Overview of skin aging and photoaging. Dermatol Nurs 2008;20(3):177–83.
102. Monheit GD, Chastain MA. Chemical peels. Facial Plast Surg Clin North Am 2001;9(2):239–55, viii.
103. Clark E, Scerri L. Superficial and medium-depth chemical peels. Clin Dermatol 2008;26(2):209–18.
104. Alexiades-Armenakas MR, Dover JS, Arndt KA. The spectrum of laser skin resurfacing: nonablative, fractional, and ablative laser resurfacing. J Am Acad Dermatol 2008;58(5):719–37.
105. Ehrlich M, Rao J, Pabby A, et al. Improvement in the appearance of wrinkles with topical transforming growth factor beta(1) and l-ascorbic acid. Dermatol Surg 2006;32(5):618–25.
106. Fitzpatrick RE, Rostan EF. Reversal of photodamage with topical growth factors: a pilot study. J Cosmet Laser Ther 2003;5(1):25–34.
107. Cass DL, Meuli M, Adzick NS. Scar wars: implications of fetal wound healing for the pediatric burn patient. Pediatr Surg Int 1997;12(7):484–9.
108. Gold MH, Goldman MP, Biron J. Efficacy of novel skin cream containing mixture of human growth factors and cytokines for skin rejuvenation. J Drugs Dermatol 2007;6(2):197–201.
109. Tajima S, Wachi H, Uemura Y, et al. Modulation by elastin peptide VGVAPG of cell proliferation and elastin expression in human skin fibroblasts. Arch Dermatol Res 1997;289(8):489–92.
110. Kamoun A, Landeau JM, Godeau G, et al. Growth stimulation of human skin fibroblasts by elastin-derived peptides. Cell Adhes Commun 1995;3(4):273–81.
111. Lintner K. Promoting production in the extracellular matrix without compromising barrier. Cutis 2002;70(Suppl 6):13–6.
112. Katayama K, Armendariz-Borunda J, Raghow R, et al. A pentapeptide from type I procollagen promotes extracellular matrix production. J Biol Chem 1993; 268(14):9941–4.
113. Robinson LR, Fitzgerald NC, Doughty DG, et al. Topical palmitoyl pentapeptide provides improvement in photoaged human facial skin. Int J Cosmet Sci 2005; 27(3):155–60.
114. Blanes-Mira C, Clemente J, Jodas G, et al. A synthetic hexapeptide (Argireline) with antiwrinkle activity. Int J Cosmet Sci 2002;24(5):303–10.
115. Pickart L, Freedman JH, Loker WJ, et al. Growth-modulating plasma tripeptide may function by facilitating copper uptake into cells. Nature 1980;288(5792): 715–7.
116. Buffoni F, Pino R, Dal PA. Effect of tripeptide-copper complexes on the process of skin wound healing and on cultured fibroblasts. Arch Int Pharmacodyn Ther 1995;330(3):345–60.

Botulinum Toxin in Facial Rejuvenation: An Update

Jean Carruthers, MD[a],*, Alastair Carruthers, MD[b]

KEYWORDS

- Botox • Rejuvenation • Facial reshaping • Adjunctive uses
- Safety • Predictability

Since its initial approval by the US Food and Drug Administration (FDA) 20 years ago for the treatment of strabismus, hemifacial spasm, and blepharospasm in adults, botulinum toxin (BTX) has become one of the most frequently requested products in cosmetic rejuvenation around the world. After years of clinical success and consistent safety in the upper face, the use of BTX has expanded and evolved to include increasingly complicated indications. In the hands of adept injectors, the focus has shifted from the treatment of individual dynamic rhytides to shaping, contouring, and sculpting, alone or in combination with other cosmetic procedures, to enhance the aesthetic appearance of the face. Although recent reports have questioned the safety of BTX, 25 years of therapeutic and over 20 years of cosmetic use has demonstrated an impressive record of safety and efficacy when used appropriately by experienced injectors.

HISTORY AND CLINICAL DEVELOPMENT

First identified well over 100 years ago as a cause of food poisoning, the bacterium *Clostridium botulinum* was studied extensively over the next 50 years, leading to the identification of seven distinct serotypes, and the isolation and purification of BTX type A (BTX-A).[1,2] In 1980s, Scott published the landmark paper establishing the safety of BTX-A in humans for the treatment of strabismus.[3] In 1987, Carruthers and Carruthers noticed that patients treated for blepharospasm also experienced an improvement in glabellar rhytides; the subsequent publication of their results[4] sparked a flurry of interest and additional studies.[5,6] Since then, BTX-A has been approved by the FDA for a variety of applications, including strabismus, blepharospasm, cervical

This article originally appeared in *Dermatologic Clinics* 2009;27(4):417–425.

[a] Department of Ophthalmology and Visual Sciences, University of British Columbia, 943 West Broadway, Suite 740, Vancouver, BC, Canada V5Z 4E1

[b] Department of Dermatology and Skin Science, University of British Columbia, 943 West Broadway, Suite 820, Vancoucer, BC, Canada V5Z 4E1

* Corresponding author.

E-mail address: drjean@carruthers.net

doi:10.1016/j.ogc.2010.10.002
0889-8545/10/$ – see front matter © 2010 Elsevier Inc. All rights reserved.
obgyn.theclinics.com

dystonia, hyperhidrosis, and mild-to-moderate glabellar rhytides, and by Health Canada for facial wrinkling.

FORMULATIONS

The majority of peer-reviewed reports in the literature focus on the original formulation of BTX-A: BOTOX Cosmetic (Vistabel in most of Europe and Vistabex in Italy; Allergan, Inc, Irvine, CA, USA). BOTOX has been approved for 20 indications in more than 75 countries.[7] However, several other products are or will be available in the near future. Reloxin (Dysport; Ipsen Ltd, United Kingdom/Medicis, Scottsdale, AZ, USA) is expected to receive FDA approval for cosmetic applications in North America in April 2009 and has already received approval in 15 European countries as Azzalure (Galderma, France). Its UK counterpart, Dysport, is approved in over 65 countries for therapeutic indications and differs from BOTOX in purification procedures.[8] There is some evidence that Dysport may show greater diffusion and migration, with increased potential for side effects and less precise localization of clinical effects.[9–11] Dose ratios between Dysport and BOTOX have ranged in the literature from 6:1 to 1:1, though new evidence suggests a more suitable dose ratio of less than 3:1.[12,13]

Xeomin (NT-201; Merz Pharmaceuticals, Frankfurt, Germany) is the third BTX-A licensed in Germany. It has received approval for the treatment of blepharospasm and cervical dystonia in some European countries, Mexico, and Argentina; for glabellar rhytides in Argentina; and is in Phase 3 testing for glabellar lines in North America.[8] In potency, Xeomin appears to exhibit a 1:1 dose ratio when compared with BOTOX,[14] and therapeutic clinical studies have found similar levels of efficacy and safety.[15,16] Xeomin is free of complexing proteins, which some believe may result in purer formulations with greater efficacy and a reduced risk of sensitization and antibody formation.[16]

The only available BTX type B in North America and Europe, Myobloc/NeuroBloc (Solstice Neurosciences Inc/Eisai Co, Ltd) is approved for the treatment of cervical dystonia.[8] Clinical data indicate that injections of Myobloc for cosmetic applications are more painful with a shorter duration of effect,[17,18] but are associated with a more rapid onset of action and a greater area of diffusion.[19]

PureTox (Mentor Corp, Santa Barbara, CA, USA) is an uncomplexed type A neurotoxin, similar to Xeomin, in Phase 3 testing for glabellar rhytides, and in various stages of development for therapeutic indications in the United States. Globally, several other BTX products are under development.[8] Chinese BTX-A (CBTX-A; marketed as Prosigne in Brazil; Lanzhou Institute of Biological Products, China) is the only approved BTX-A in China, contains bovine gelatin protein, and appears to be slightly less effective than BOTOX.[20] CBTX-A must be distinguished from CNBTX-A (Nanfeng Medical Science and Technology Development Co, Ltd), which is neither licensed nor approved in any country and contains significantly higher levels of BTX, despite appearances to the contrary when it is sold by way of the Internet. The high levels of BTX may constitute a severe health risk for patients.[21] Neuronox (Medy-Tox Inc, South Korea) is widely used in Korea and Southeast Asia. Little has been published about Neuronox, although Stone and colleagues report that Neuronox and BOTOX produce equivalent responses in a murine model.[22]

COSMETIC APPLICATIONS OF BOTULINUM TOXIN-A

Since the initial FDA approval of BTX-A for therapeutic applications, practitioners have employed the neurotoxin to treat a variety of hyperkinetic facial lines, including crow's feet, horizontal forehead lines and glabellar rhytides in the upper face (**Figs. 1–3**) and

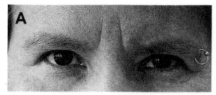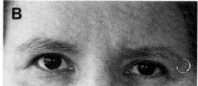

Fig. 1. Cosmetic use of BTX-A in the upper face: (*A*) prior to injection (*B*) and after treatment for glabellar lines, crow's feet, and horizontal forehead rhytides.

folds and lines in the lower face and neck (see **Fig. 3**; **Figs. 4–7**), with a high level of efficacy and patient satisfaction.[23–28] As injector and recipient confidence has grown, so too have the areas of application; now, BTX-A is used to sculpt the face and restore symmetry, and is a useful adjunct to other cosmetic applications and surgery.

Facial Sculpting

In the upper face, BTX-A is capable of lifting the brow and widening the eyes. Several reports noted that injections in the glabella resulted in central, medial, and lateral brow elevation,[29–31] which has been shown to be the result of partial inactivation and increased resting tone of the frontalis.[31] Similarly, small doses of BTX-A injected into the lower pretarsal orbicularis open the palpebral aperture at rest and at smile in individuals who desire a wider, rounder eye.[32,33] In the lower face, BTX injections into the masseter can alter the shape of the jawline and has been well documented in East Asian populations, with up to 50% reduction in muscle thickness and bulk.[34–37] More recently, the toxin has been shown to be beneficial in improving the aesthetic appearance of the face in non-Asian populations.[38,39] Liew and Dart investigated the use of BTX for aesthetic reshaping of the mandibular angle in a Western population compared with an East Asian control group.[38] While all patients achieved aesthetic improvement of the shape of their lower face, aesthetic improvement in Western patients was achieved with smaller doses of BTX-A (25–30 U) compared to doses required in the East Asian control group (40 U), and the effects lasted for 9 to 12 months. Moreover, Western patients experienced additional improvement in function attributed to bruxism, an effect that has been noted elsewhere in the literature,[40] lasting for 6 to 7 months.

Adjunctive Botulinum Toxin-A

BTX-A is used increasingly in combination with other cosmetic procedures to prolong and enhance aesthetic results. The combination of BTX-A and soft-tissue

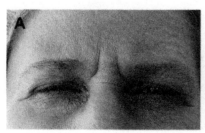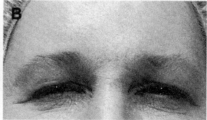

Fig. 2. Glabella before (*A*) and after (*B*) combined treatment with BTX-A and hyaluronic acid.

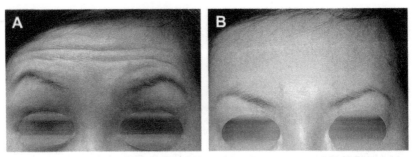

Fig. 3. Horizontal forehead lines before (A) and after (B) treatment with BTX-A.

augmentation is a highly synergistic approach used to achieve more effective, longer-lasting results by reducing the dynamic component of the target rhytide, especially when used in the glabella, brow, forehead, zygomatic and perioral regions, and in the neck.[41–44] Combination therapy leads to greater patients' satisfaction and superior efficacy compared with fillers alone (see **Fig. 3**).[43,45,46] Similarly, the benefits of laser resurfacing can be optimized by pretreatment with BTX-A, leading to superior and longer-lasting aesthetic outcomes.[42,47–49] Studies of Intense Pulsed Light show that combination therapy with BTX-A increases the overall aesthetic benefit and improves skin texture and the appearance of telangiectasias (see **Figs. 4** and **5**).[50,51]

Finally, many cosmetic surgeons consider BTX-A a key adjunct in surgical interventions; the neurotoxin serves to increase longevity of the procedure and aids in wound healing by reducing repetitive muscular actions that can hasten dehiscence.[42,47] Indeed, multiple trials have shown the benefit of BTX-A injections to facilitate wound healing; pretreating the underlying musculature with BTX-A allows for the use of finer sutures and minimizes scarring by reducing tension on the wound edge, allowing it to heal more readily (**Fig. 8**).[52–54]

SAFETY

Most side effects associated with the cosmetic application of BTX-A are mild and transient and include bruising, swelling, pain around the injection site, headache, and flu like symptoms.[55] More serious complications, such as brow or eyelid ptosis, can occur but are usually associated with poor injection technique and lack of injector experience and result from diffusion of the toxin into adjacent musculature.[56]

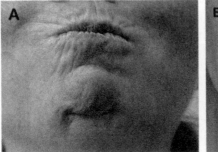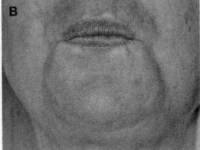

Fig. 4. Mental scar and mentalis muscle disinsertion before (A) and after (B) treatment with BTX-A.

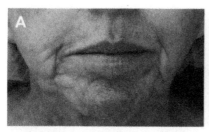
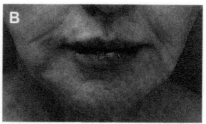

Fig. 5. Combination therapy in the lower face: before (*A*) and after treatment with BTX-A and hyaluronic acid (*B*).

Clinical Safety Profile of Botulinum Toxin

Examination of nearly 20 years of research reveals an impressive record of safety and efficacy. Most reported adverse events (AE) are transient and mild. Coté and colleagues analyzed 995 cases of nonserious side effects among 1031 AE reports submitted to the FDA; side effects included lack of intended cosmetic effect (63%), injection-site reaction (19%), ptosis (11%), muscle weakness (5%), and headache (5%).[57] Zagui and colleagues analyzed eight randomized trials and 13 case reports of cosmetic BTX up to September of 2007.[58] Of 1003 subjects, 182 (18.14%) experienced AE, of which eyelid ptosis was the most frequent (3.39%). Other side effects included headache, local reaction, and infection.

Long-term safety of multiple-injection sessions over time has been established by several analyses. Hsiung and colleagues examined 235 patients who received BTX-A injections for movement disorders over a 10-year period and found mostly minor AE in 27% of subjects.[59] Likewise, a review of 36 randomized trials and 1425 subjects who received BTX-A for therapeutic indications revealed no serious AE,[60] and the authors' own retrospective analysis of 853 upper-face treatment sessions in 50 subjects, for an average of 5.95 years, showed only 9 subjects reported AE, all transient and mild to moderate in severity, 5 of which were probably or definitely related to treatment.[61]

Indeed, research suggests that the risk of AE diminishes over multiple treatment sessions. In a multicenter study of 65 subjects who received regular BTX-A injections

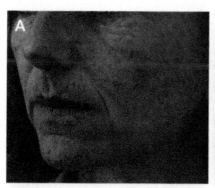
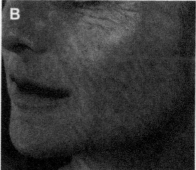

Fig. 6. Before (*A*) and after whole-face treatment with Intense Pulsed Light, BTX-A into the depressor anguli oris, mentalis, and orbicularis, plus concomitant treatment with soft-tissue augmentation of the melolabial, nasolabial, and malar regions (*B*).

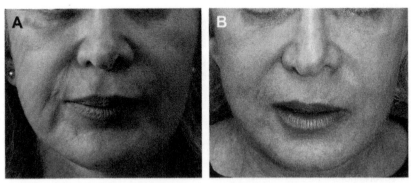

Fig. 7. Before (*A*) and after whole-face treatment with Intense Pulsed Light, BTX-A into the depressor anguli oris, mentalis, and orbicularis oris, and soft-tissue augmentation of the nasojugal folds, malar fat pads, nasolabial folds, melomental folds, and chin (*B*).

for hemifacial spasm over 10 years, Defazio and colleagues found that the incidence of AE decreased over time, falling from 37% during the first year of treatment to 12% in the tenth year.[62] In an analysis of 45 women who received continuous BTX-A injections for movement disorders for a mean duration of 15 years, recorded AE occurred in 35.6% and 22.2% of subjects at first and last visits, respectively.[63] Finally, Rzany and colleagues analyzed more than 4000 treatments in 945 people injected in the upper face and found only mild or moderate side effects, such as bruising and eyelid drooping, and side effects decreased with repeated injections.[64]

Complications

BTX works through temporary chemodenervation of the muscle, resulting in localized reduction of muscular activity. The authors believe that many complications can be

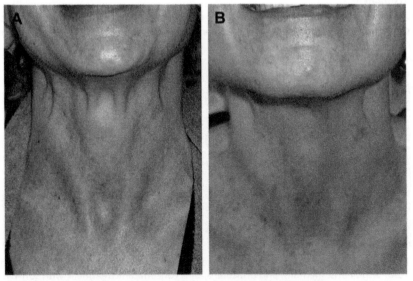

Fig. 8. Before (*A*) and after treatment of the platysma with BTX-A (*B*).

avoided by using more concentrated doses, which allows for more accurate placement of BTX, less diffusion, and greater duration of effect.

Brow and eyelid ptosis lasting for up to 3 months are the most troublesome complications that can occur in the upper face, and both are caused by diffusion of the toxin into adjacent musculature. The risk of brow ptosis, which is caused by product diffusion into the frontalis, can be avoided by preinjecting the brow depressors, avoiding preexisting brow ptosis, and injecting the glabella and forehead in separate treatment sessions.[56] Similarly, eyelid ptosis occurs when BTX-A injections into the glabella affect the upper eyelid levator muscle by way of diffusion. Higher concentrations, careful placement of the toxin (1 cm above the bony orbital rim, 1.5 cm lateral to the lateral canthus), and advising patients to refrain from manipulating the treated area for several hours after injection can help avoid eyelid ptosis. Other complications that have been reported include cocked eyebrow, diplopia, ectropion, asymmetrical smile, decreased strength of eye closure, and dry eye.[56]

In the lower face, complications are usually caused by overenthusiastic use of large doses, and can include mouth incompetence, asymmetry, drooling, difficulties in speech, and the inability to purse the lips.[56] Small doses of BTX-A injected superficially and symmetrically can decrease the potential for complications, as can placement; injections too close to the mouth or directly into the mental fold or orbicularis oris are more likely to result in undesirable effects (eg, flaccid cheek, incompetent mouth, or asymmetric smile). In the neck, large doses of BTX-A can lead to difficulty swallowing and general weakness.

Immunogenicity and Allergic Response

Antibody formation rarely occurs in current lots of BTX-A, which contain lower total protein loads than earlier formulations (prior to 1998), but has been reported, particularly when large doses are injected (eg, those associated with therapeutic applications).[63,65] Although the overall risk of antibody formation is low when using the lowest possible dose with the longest feasible intervals between injections,[66] a recent report describes an unusual case of a 20-year-old patient who developed antibody-induced therapy failure after the fourth injection series in the frontalis (60 U per session, 4 to 5 months between treatments).[67] Circulating antibodies against BTX-A were detected by indirect enzyme-linked immunosorbent assay and mouse protection assay.

Similarly, allergic reaction to BTX-A is rare but can be found in the literature. Reported reactions include serious or nonserious rashes[57,68] and granulomas.[69] Other allergic responses include a localized anaphylactic reaction in one leg,[68] a case of anaphylaxis after injection of BTX-A and lidocaine for the treatment of chronic neck and back pain,[70] and one patient who experienced severe respiratory failure after leg injections of 300 U BTX-A.[71]

Serious Adverse Events: Therapeutic Botulinum Toxin-A

A large examination of 1031 AE reports submitted to the FDA revealed 36 classified as serious for cosmetic BTX-A (headaches, facial paralysis, muscle weakness, dysphagia, flu like symptoms, and allergic reactions).[57] Of those 36, 13 had underlying disease that may have contributed to the reported AE, and serious AE were most common with significantly higher doses associated with therapeutic BTX-A. Indeed, the 407 AE reported to the FDA for the therapeutic use of BTX-A (median dose, 100 U) included 28 deaths and other serious AE, such as arrhythmia and myocardial infarction. However, the report could not determine a causal relationship between the fatalities and BTX-A injections, especially since 26 patients who died had underlying cardiovascular diseases with an elevated risk of mortality. No deaths or cardiovascular complications were reported after treatment with significantly lower cosmetic doses.

In early 2008, the national consumer advocacy group, Public Citizen, petitioned the FDA to warn the public about serious side effects associated with BTX after analyzing FDA data that included 658 AE, of which 180 were aspiration, dysphagia, or pneumonia.[72] There were 16 deaths reported, 4 of which occurred in children under the age of 18. In response, the FDA announced a pending safety review focusing on high-dose therapeutic uses of BTX.[73] The review involves a small number of AE reports and large doses in patients with juvenile cerebral palsy and other lower-limb spasticities; none of the AE relate to a death as a result of cosmetic BTX-A.

Other reports have called the safety of BTX-A into question. Media announcements of death or paralysis after injection of cosmetic BTX-A were ultimately found to be the result of fake products that are unapproved, untested, and of questionable content.[74,75] In 2008, Antonucci and colleagues[76] injected BTX-A into the whisker muscles of rats and mice and found trace amounts of the toxin in the brainstem three days later. However, the BTX-A used in the study was an uncomplexed toxin (150,000 kDa molecule) produced in the laboratory for veterinarian research purposes and is not approved for human use by any governing body, and the doses used were up to 10 times higher than approved doses to treat glabellar rhytides in humans (translating into up to 150 times higher per kilogram/body weight).

SUMMARY

Botulinum toxins have been used therapeutically in humans for nearly 30 years and carry an impressive record of efficacy and safety when used appropriately. Originally used for the treatment of simple rhytides in the upper face, BTX-A is used to sculpt and mould the face into more pleasing contours, and is now considered an integral component of facial rejuvenation and an adjunct to other cosmetic surgical and nonsurgical procedures. Side effects are mostly mild and transient; more serious complications and AE are caused by poor injection technique or doses that are too large in already medically compromised patients. With the tiny amounts of BTX used for cosmetic applications, complications are usually local and related to injection technique. In addition, systemic complications virtually never occur because of the smaller doses necessary for cosmetic applications. Careful adherence to product, dosing, and placement can do much for the avoidance of more serious AE. Indeed, it is the authors' prediction that the uses of BTX and development of new products will only continue to grow in the next few years.

REFERENCES

1. Schantz EJ. Historical perspective. In: Jankovic J, Hallet M, editors. Therapy with botulinum toxin. New York: Marcel Dekker Inc; 1994.
2. Schantz EJ, Johnson EA. Preparation and characterization of botulinum toxin type A for human treatment. In: Jankovic J, Hallet M, editors. Therapy with botulinum toxin. New York: Marcel Dekker Inc; 1994.
3. Scott AB. Botulinum toxin injection into extraocular muscles as an alternative to strabismus surgery. Ophthalmology 1980;87:1044–9.
4. Carruthers JDA, Carruthers JA. Treatment of glabellar frown lines with C. Botulinum A exotoxin. J Dermatol Surg Oncol 1992;18:17–21.
5. Borodic GE, Cheney M, McKenna M. Contralateral injections of botulinum A toxin for the treatment of hemifacial spasm to achieve increased facial symmetry. Plast Reconstr Surg 1992;90:972–7.

6. Blitzer A, Brin MF, Keen MS, et al. Botulinum toxin for the treatment of hyperfunctional lines of the face. Arch Otolaryngol Head Neck Surg 1993;119:1018–22.
7. Carruthers J, Carruthers A. The evolution of botulinum neurotoxin type A for cosmetic applications. J Cosmet Laser Ther 2007;9:186–92.
8. Carruthers A, Carruthers J. Botulinum toxin products overview. Skin Therapy Lett 2008;13:1–4.
9. Lowe PL, Patnaik R, Lowe NJ. A comparison of two botulinum type A toxin preparations for the treatment of glabellar lines: double-blind, randomized, pilot study. Dermatol Surg 2005;31:1651–4.
10. Trindade de Almeida AR, Marques E, de Almeida J, et al. Pilot study comparing the diffusion of two formulations of botulinum toxin type A in patients with forehead hyperhidrosis. Dermatol Surg 2007;33(1 Spec No):S37–43.
11. Cliff SH, Judodihardjo H, Eltringham E. Different formulations of botulinum toxin type A have different migration characteristics: a double-blind, randomized study. J Cosmet Dermatol 2008;7:50–4.
12. Karsai S, Raulin C. Current evidence on the unit equivalence of different botulinum neurotoxin A formulations and recommendations for clinical practice in dermatology. Dermatol Surg 2009;35:1–8.
13. Kranz G, Haubenberger D, Voller B, et al. Respective potencies of Botox(R) and Dysport(R) in a human skin model: a randomized, double-blind study. Mov Disord 2009;24:231–6.
14. Dressler D. [Pharmacological aspects of therapeutic botulinum toxin preparations]. Nervenarzt 2006;77:912–21 [in German].
15. Roggenkamper P, Jost WH, Bihari K, et al. Efficacy and safety of a new botulinum toxin type A free of complexing proteins in the treatment of blepharospasm. J Neural Transm 2006;113:303–12.
16. Jost WH, Blumel J, Grafe S. Botulinum neurotoxin type A free of complexing proteins (XEOMIN) in focal dystonia. Drugs 2007;67:669–83.
17. Spencer JM, Gordon M, Goldberg DJ. Botulinum B treatment of the glabellar and frontalis regions: a dose response analysis. J Cosmet Laser Ther 2002;4:19–23.
18. Jacob CI. Botulinum neurotoxin type B–a rapid wrinkle reducer. Semin Cutan Med Surg 2003;22:131–5.
19. Flynn TC, Clark RE. Botulinum toxin type B (MYOBLOC) versus botulinum type A (BOTOX) frontalis study: rate of onset and radius of diffusion. Dermatol Surg 2003;29:519–22.
20. Tang X, Wan X. Comparison of botox with a Chinese type A botulinum toxin. Chin Med J 2000;113:794–8.
21. Hunt T, Clarke K. Potency of the botulinum toxin product CNBTX-A significantly exceeds labeled units in standard potency test. J Am Acad Dermatol 2008;58:517–8.
22. Stone AV, Ma J, Whitlock PW, et al. Effects of botox and neuronox on muscle force generation in mice. J Orthop Res 2007;25:1658–64.
23. Carruthers A, Carruthers J. Botulinum toxin type A: history and current cosmetic use in the upper face. Semin Cutan Med Surg 2001;20:71–84.
24. Carruthers J, Carruthers A. Botulinum toxin A in the mid and lower face and neck. Dermatol Clin 2004;22:151–8.
25. Lowe NJ, Yamauchi P. Cosmetic uses of botulinum toxins for lower aspects of the face and neck. Clin Dermatol 2004;22:18–22.
26. Dayan SH, Maas CS. Botulinum toxins for facial wrinkles: beyond glabellar lines. Facial Plast Surg Clin North Am 2007;15:41–9.

27. Kaplan SE, Sherris DA, Gassner HG, et al. The use of botulinum toxin A in perioral rejuvenation. Facial Plast Surg Clin North Am 2007;15:415–21.
28. Fagien S, Carruthers JD. A comprehensive review of patient-reported satisfaction with botulinum toxin type a for aesthetic procedures. Plast Reconstr Surg 2008; 122:1915–25.
29. Frankel AS, Kamer FM. Chemical browlift. Arch Otolaryngol Head Neck Surg 1998;124:321–3.
30. Huilgol S, Carruthers JA, Carruthers JDA. Raising eyebrows with botulinum toxin. Dermatol Surg 1999;25:373–6.
31. Carruthers A, Carruthers J. Eyebrow height after botulinum toxin type A to the glabella. Dermatol Surg 2007;33:26–32.
32. Flynn TC, Carruthers JA, Carruthers JA. Botulinum-A toxin treatment of the lower eyelid improves infraorbital rhytides and widens the eye. Dermatol Surg 2001;27: 703–8.
33. Flynn TC, Carruthers JA, Carruthers JA, et al. Botulinum A toxin (BOTOX) in the lower eyelid: dose-finding study. Dermatol Surg 2003;29:943–50.
34. To EW, Ahuja AT, Ho WS, et al. A prospective study of the effect of botulinum toxin A on masseteric muscle hypertrophy with ultrasonographic and electromyographic measurement. Br J Plast Surg 2001;54:197–200.
35. von Lindern JJ, Niederhagen B, Appel T, et al. Type A botulinum toxin for the treatment of hypertrophy of the masseter and temporal muscle: an alternative treatment. Plast Reconstr Surg 2001;107:327–32.
36. Park MY, Ahn KY, Jung DS. Application of botulinum toxin A for treatment of facial contouring in the lower face. Dermatol Surg 2003;29:477–83.
37. Kim NH, Chung JH, Park RH, et al. The use of botulinum toxin type A in aesthetic mandibular contouring. Plast Reconstr Surg 2005;115:919–30.
38. Liew S, Dart A. Nonsurgical reshaping of the lower face. Aesthet Surg J 2008;28: 251–7.
39. Tartaro G, Rauso R, Santagata M, et al. Lower facial contouring with botulinum toxin type A. J Craniofac Surg 2008;19:1613–7.
40. Chikhani L, Dichamp J. [Bruxism, temporo-mandibular dysfunction and botulinum toxin]. Ann Readapt Med Phys 2003;46:333–7 [in French].
41. Fagien S. Botox for the treatment of dynamic and hyperkinetic facial lines and furrows: adjunctive use in facial aesthetic surgery. Plast Reconstr Surg 1999; 103:701–13.
42. Fagien S, Brandt FS. Primary and adjunctive use of botulinum toxin type A (botox) in facial aesthetic surgery: beyond the glabella. Clin Plast Surg 2001;28:127–48.
43. Carruthers J, Carruthers A. A prospective, randomized, parallel group study analyzing the effect of BTX-A(botox) and nonanimal sourced hyaluronic acid (NASHA, restylane) in combination compared with NASHA (restylane) alone in severe glabellar rhytides in adult female subjects: treatment of severe glabellar rhytides with a hyaluronic acid derivative compared with the derivative and BTX-A. Dermatol Surg 2003;29:802–9.
44. Coleman KR, Carruthers J. Combination therapy with BOTOX and fillers: the new rejuvenation paradigm. Dermatol Ther 2006;19:177–88.
45. Carruthers J, Carruthers A, Maberley D. Deep resting glabellar rhytides respond to BTX-A and Hylan B. Dermatol Surg 2003;29:539–44.
46. Patel MP, Talmor M, Nolan WB. Botox and collagen for glabellar furrows: advantages of combination therapy. Ann Plast Surg 2004;52:442–7.
47. Carruthers J, Carruthers A. The adjunctive usage of botulinum. Dermatol Surg 1998;24:1244–7.

48. West TB, Alster TS. Effect of botulinum toxin type A on movement-associated rhytides following CO_2 laser resurfacing. Dermatol Surg 1999;25:259–61.
49. Zimbler MS, Holds JB, Kokoska MS, et al. Effect of botulinum toxin pretreatment on laser resurfacing results: a prospective, randomized, blinded trial. Arch Facial Plast Surg 2001;3:165–9.
50. Carruthers J, Carruthers A. The effect of full-face broadband light treatments alone and in combination with bilateral crow's feet botulinum toxin type A chemodenervation. Dermatol Surg 2004;30:355–66.
51. Khoury JG, Saluja R, Goldman MP. The effect of botulinum toxin type A on full-face intense pulsed light treatment: a randomized, double-blind, split-face study. Dermatol Surg 2008;34:1062–9.
52. Sherris DA, Gassner HG. Botulinum toxin to minimize facial scarring. Facial Plast Surg 2002;18:35–9.
53. Gassner HG, Brissett AE, Otley CC, et al. Botulinum toxin to improve facial wound healing: a prospective, blinded, placebo-controlled study. Mayo Clin Proc 2006; 81:1023–8.
54. Wilson AM. Use of botulinum toxin type A to prevent widening of facial scars. Plast Reconstr Surg 2006;117:1758–66.
55. Alam M, Dover JS, Klein AW, et al. Botulinum A exotoxin for hyperfunctional facial lines: where not to inject. Arch Dermatol 2002;138:1180.
56. Klein AW. Complications, adverse reactions, and insights with the use of botulinum toxin. Dermatol Surg 2003;29:549–56.
57. Coté TR, Mohan AK, Polder JA, et al. Botulinum toxin type A injections: adverse events reported to the US Food and Drug Administration in therapeutic and cosmetic cases. J Am Acad Dermatol 2005;53:407–15.
58. Zagui RM, Matayoshi S, Moura FC. [Adverse effects associated with facial application of botulinum toxin: a systematic review with meta-analysis]. Arq Bras Oftalmol 2008;71:894–901 [in Portuguese].
59. Hsiung GY, Das SK, Ranawaya R, et al. Long-term efficacy of botulinum toxin A in treatment of various movement disorders over a 10-year period. Mov Disord 2002;17:1288–93.
60. Naumann M, Jankovic J. Safety of botulinum toxin type A: a systematic review and meta-analysis. Curr Med Res Opin 2004;20:981–90.
61. Carruthers J, Carruthers A. Complications of botulinum toxin A. Facial Plast Surg Clin North Am 2007;15:51–4.
62. Defazio G, Abbruzzese G, Girlanda P, et al. Botulinum toxin A treatment for primary hemifacial spasm: a 10-year multicenter study. Arch Neurol 2002;59:418–20.
63. Mejia NI, Vuong KD, Jankovic J. Long-term botulinum toxin efficacy, safety, and immunogenicity. Mov Disord 2005;20:592–7.
64. Rzany B, Dill-Müller D, Grablowitz D, et al. Repeated botulinum toxin A injections for the treatment of lines in the upper face: a retrospective study of 4,103 treatments in 945 patients. Dermatol Surg 2007;33(1 Spec No):S18–25.
65. Jankovic J, Vuong KD, Ahsan J. Comparison of efficacy and immunogenicity of original versus current botulinum toxin in cervical dystonia. Neurology 2003;60: 1186–8.
66. Allergan, Inc. Botox cosmetic (botulinum toxin type A) purified neurotoxin complex (prescribing information). Irvine (CA): Allergan, Inc; 2005.
67. Lee SK. Antibody-induced failure of botulinum toxin type A therapy in a patient with masseteric hypertrophy. Dermatol Surg 2007;33(1 Spec No):S105–10.
68. LeWitt PA, Trosch RM. Idiosyncratic adverse reactions to intramuscular botulinum toxin type A injection. Mov Disord 1997 Nov;12:1064–7.

69. Ahbib S, Lachapelle JM, Marot L. [Sarcoidal granulomas following injections of botulic toxin A (Botox) for corrections of wrinkles]. Ann Dermatol Venereol 2006;133:43–5 [in French].
70. Li M, Goldberger BA, Hopkins C. Fatal case of BOTOX-related anaphylaxis? J Forensic Sci 2005;50:169–72.
71. Nong LB, He WQ, Xu YH, et al. [Severe respiratory failure after injection of botulinum toxin: case report and review of the literature]. Zhonghua Jie He He Hu Xi Za Zhi 2008;31:369–71 [in Chinese].
72. Public Citizen. Stricter warnings needed for botox, myobloc injections. Available at: http://www.citizen.org/pressroom/release.cfm?ID=2593. Accessed February 6, 2009.
73. U.S. Food and Drug Administration. Early communication about an ongoing safety review botox and botox cosmetic (botulinum toxin type A) and myobloc (botulinum toxin type B). Plast Surg Nurs 2008;28:150–1.
74. USA TODAY 219 doctors purchase Botox knockoff. Available at: http://www.usatoday.com/news/health/2005-02-21-fake-botox-usat_x.htm. Accessed February 6, 2009.
75. The Business Edition. Woman dies from fake Botox injections. Available at: http://www.thebusinessedition.com/woman-dies-from-fake-botox-injections-213/#more-213. Accessed February 6, 2009.
76. Antonucci F, Rossi C, Gianfranceschi L, et al. Long-distance retrograde effects of botulinum neurotoxin A. J Neurosci 2008;28:3689–96.

Index

Note: Page numbers of article titles are in **boldface** type.

Obstet Gynecol Clin N Am 37 (2010) 583–589
doi:10.1016/S0889-8545(10)00105-1
0889-8545/10/$ – see front matter © 2010 Elsevier Inc. All rights reserved.

obgyn.theclinics.com

Moving?

Make sure your subscription moves with you!

To notify us of your new address, find your **Clinics Account Number** (located on your mailing label above your name), and contact customer service at:

Email: journalscustomerservice-usa@elsevier.com

800-654-2452 (subscribers in the U.S. & Canada)
314-447-8871 (subscribers outside of the U.S. & Canada)

Fax number: 314-447-8029

Elsevier Health Sciences Division
Subscription Customer Service
3251 Riverport Lane
Maryland Heights, MO 63043

*To ensure uninterrupted delivery of your subscription,
please notify us at least 4 weeks in advance of move.

United States Postal Service

Statement of Ownership, Management, and Circulation
(All Periodicals Publications Except Requestor Publications)

1. Publication Title	2. Publication Number							3. Filing Date
Obstetrics and Gynecology Clinics of North America	0	0	0	-	2	7	6	9/15/10

4. Issue Frequency	5. Number of Issues Published Annually	6. Annual Subscription Price
Mar, Jun, Sep, Dec	4	$257.00

7. Complete Mailing Address of Known Office of Publication (Not printer) (Street, city, county, state, and ZIP+4®)

Elsevier Inc.
360 Park Avenue South
New York, NY 10010-1710

Contact Person
Stephen Bushing
Telephone (Include area code)
215-239-3688

8. Complete Mailing Address of Headquarters or General Business Office of Publisher (Not printer)

Elsevier Inc., 360 Park Avenue South, New York, NY 10010-1710

9. Full Names and Complete Mailing Addresses of Publisher, Editor, and Managing Editor (Do not leave blank)

Publisher (Name and complete mailing address)

Kim Murphy, Elsevier, Inc., 1600 John F. Kennedy Blvd. Suite 1800, Philadelphia, PA 19103-2899

Editor (Name and complete mailing address)

Carla Holloway, Elsevier, Inc., 1600 John F. Kennedy Blvd. Suite 1800, Philadelphia, PA 19103-2899

Managing Editor (Name and complete mailing address)

Catherine Bewick, Elsevier, Inc., 1600 John F. Kennedy Blvd. Suite 1800, Philadelphia, PA 19103-2899

10. Owner (Do not leave blank. If the publication is owned by a corporation, give the name and address of the corporation immediately followed by the names and addresses of all stockholders owning or holding 1 percent or more of the total amount of stock. If not owned by a corporation, give the names and addresses of the individual owners. If owned by a partnership or other unincorporated firm, give its name and address as well as those of each individual owner. If the publication is published by a nonprofit organization, give its name and address.)

Full Name	Complete Mailing Address
Wholly owned subsidiary of	4520 East-West Highway
Reed/Elsevier, US holdings	Bethesda, MD 20814

11. Known Bondholders, Mortgagees, and Other Security Holders Owning or Holding 1 Percent or More of Total Amount of Bonds, Mortgages, or Other Securities. If none, check box ☐ None

Full Name	Complete Mailing Address
N/A	

12. Tax Status (For completion by nonprofit organizations authorized to mail at nonprofit rates) (Check one)
The purpose, function, and nonprofit status of this organization and the exempt status for federal income tax purposes:
☐ Has Not Changed During Preceding 12 Months
☐ Has Changed During Preceding 12 Months (Publisher must submit explanation of change with this statement)

PS Form 3526, September 2007 (Page 1 of 3 (Instructions Page 3)) PSN 7530-01-000-9931 PRIVACY NOTICE: See our Privacy policy in www.usps.com

13. Publication Title		14. Issue Date for Circulation Data Below
Obstetrics and Gynecology Clinics of North America		September 2010

15. Extent and Nature of Circulation		Average No. Copies Each Issue During Preceding 12 Months	No. Copies of Single Issue Published Nearest to Filing Date
a. Total Number of Copies (Net press run)		1574	1492
b. Paid Circulation (By Mail and Outside the Mail)	(1) Mailed Outside-County Paid Subscriptions Stated on PS Form 3541. (Include paid distribution above nominal rate, advertiser's proof copies, and exchange copies)	490	440
	(2) Mailed In-County Paid Subscriptions Stated on PS Form 3541 (Include paid distribution above nominal rate, advertiser's proof copies, and exchange copies)		
	(3) Paid Distribution Outside the Mails Including Sales Through Dealers and Carriers, Street Vendors, Counter Sales, and Other Paid Distribution Outside USPS®	507	478
	(4) Paid Distribution by Other Classes Mailed Through the USPS (e.g. First-Class Mail®)		
c. Total Paid Distribution (Sum of 15b (1), (2), (3), and (4)) ▶		997	918
d. Free or Nominal Rate Distribution (By Mail and Outside the Mail)	(1) Free or Nominal Rate Outside-County Copies Included on PS Form 3541	106	78
	(2) Free or Nominal Rate In-County Copies Included on PS Form 3541		
	(3) Free or Nominal Rate Copies Mailed at Other Classes Through the USPS (e.g. First-Class Mail)		
	(4) Free or Nominal Rate Distribution Outside the Mail (Carriers or other means)		
e. Total Free or Nominal Rate Distribution (Sum of 15d (1), (2), (3) and (4)) ▶		106	78
f. Total Distribution (Sum of 15c and 15e) ▶		1103	996
g. Copies not Distributed (See instructions to publishers #4 (page #3)) ▶		471	496
h. Total (Sum of 15f and g) ▶		1574	1492
i. Percent Paid (15c divided by 15f times 100) ▶		90.39%	92.17%

16. Publication of Statement of Ownership

☐ If the publication is a general publication, publication of this statement is required. Will be printed in the December 2010 issue of this publication. ☐ Publication not required

17. Signature and Title of Editor, Publisher, Business Manager, or Owner

Stephen R. Bushing

Stephen R. Bushing – Fulfillment/Inventory Specialist

Date: September 15, 2010

I certify that all information furnished on this form is true and complete. I understand that anyone who furnishes false or misleading information on this form or who omits material or information requested on the form may be subject to criminal sanctions (including fines and imprisonment) and/or civil sanctions (including civil penalties).

PS Form 3526, September 2007 (Page 2 of 3)